MW00605030

To Courtney,
Best wishes for good
health and a long and
productive life
PR Baker

# LIVING HEALTHY AND LOVING LIFE

# LIVING HEALTHY AND LOVING LIFE

Maurice Baker M.D.

Salt Lake City 2014

© 2014 by Maurice Baker M.D.

All rights reserved. No part of this book may be reproduced by any means, electronic or mechanical, by any information storage and retrieval system, without permission in writing from the publisher.

Printed in the United States of America

ISBN 978-0-692-29332-4

# TABLE OF CONTENTS

# ACKNOWLEDGEMENTS

My deepest appreciation to the many patients who have helped make my life complete through their confidence in my approach to their medical problems. I will forever be grateful for their example of strength and tenacity in working through their health challenges, often against seemingly impossible odds. Patients are wonderful!

Special thanks to Audrey for her meticulous efforts in making the appropriate corrections of spelling and grammar, as she read and re-read the manuscript. Also for her encouragement in writing the book.

# PREFACE

The Incas of Peru had an efficient postal service. Little huts were built along the narrow pathways and steps of a mountain. Runners trained in speed and endurance were stationed in those huts; their business was to forward government dispatches without delay. The *chasquis*, as they were called, would take verbal messages; knotted cords (*quipus*), which were their records; or even small packages and deliver them on a strict schedule. The chasquis could carry dispatches at the rate of 150 miles a day and also deliver fresh, ocean-caught fish to mountainous, land-bound Cuzco. This delivery institution was used in both Peru and Mexico long before the "civilized" nations of Europe had a postal service.

Like the chasquis, I will communicate to you mountains of information, some of which might perhaps smell like fish, it will be so old. In fact, a reference or two may be 60 or more years old—yet still valid. And some information will be nearly as fresh as the apples picked from the tree in my backyard. In all cases, rest assured that I have been accurate in my research and in the interpretation of data (our modern *quipus*), and likewise accurate in expressing my experiences and stories from my long life and decades of medical experience as a family doctor treating patients in Salt Lake City, Utah.

So, on to medicine and your health.

The American Medical Association's Code of Medical Ethics states: "The practice of medicine… is fundamentally a moral activity that arises from the imperative to care for patients and to alleviate suffering…The relationship between patient and physician is based on trust and gives rise to physicians' ethical obligation to place patients' welfare above their own self-interest… and to advocate for their patients' welfare." Fair enough. This gives us some guidelines when talking about the future of your health.

As a doctor, I feel that the first contact with each patient is critical. I believe a physician must get into the patient's heart, so to speak, before he can get into her mind. It's been my experience that an end result of trust, compliance, and reaching health goals is far more likely under these circumstances.

The encounter, then, becomes a partnership. A partnership has broad implications. In a partnership, both entities (physician and patient) negotiate with one another, coming up with agreements and common goals through a process of collaboration.

**Collaboration:** The doctor-patient relationship takes advantage of both sides of the conversation. Collaboration builds rapport (this is the "getting into the heart" approach.) The doctor has the expertise and experience to direct the therapy; the patient comes to the doctor with the motivation to make the necessary changes. Now, that motivation is often frail. This process we are addressing is focused on mutual understanding—not on the caregiver always being right. After all, "I am right and you are wrong" doesn't promote cooperation. On the other hand, the doctor doesn't have to agree with the patient if the patient clearly needs correction. From time to time, you will have to make corrections in your own quest for better health, and issues will indeed need to be addressed.

**Direction and Correction:** How is it done? The caregiver draws out the individual's own thoughts and ideas, rather than imposing his opinions. As a patient, your feelings and ideas about changes you want to make may need fine-tuning, and I hope that reading this book will provide you with both direction and correction.

**Goals:** As a reader of this book, the collaborative doctor-patient relationship is obviously more difficult because you and I won't have easy access to one another, nor a chance to negotiate what your goals will be. Your job will be to create your own lucid set of goals and keep track of them through your journey with this book.

Goals are more often achieved when the informed patient takes the initiative to create them and write them down. When you create goals, they are truly goals. When a doctor simply lists them for you, they are, instead, assignments. If they are to be reached, goals must fit your capabilities and personal vision. Unrealistic goals encourage failure and frustration. *The power for change rests within the patient.* Ultimately, it is up to you to follow through with making changes happen.

**Choices:** This may come as a little bit of a surprise, but I believe there is no single right way to change your lifestyle; instead, there are multiple options. Throughout this book, there will often, for your consideration, be several equally viable options in dietary and exercise selections. I think you will have enough information to make an educated selection that works for you. When the patient makes the choice, commitment increases.

In working with patients and constructing a plan for their treatment, I have never subscribed to the philosophy that "one size fits all." My experience is that this is not the most accurate or even the best approach. We have protocols in medicine that sometimes suggest everyone be blanketed with the same quilt. The revered evidence-based medicine approach tells us that guidelines are the best form of treatment for most patients. That would lead us to believe that our approach should be to put everyone in the same pot.

In thinking more deeply about this, let's stir this pot and see what comes to the top. The patients who succeed in rising up will do so not particularly because of what a doctor has done but because of their innate commitment—uncommon to most of us. As for those deeper down in the stew? We care for them, as well.

The caregiver helps the patient to believe in himself, rather than pointing out the fears, guilt, and failures of previous attempts to change. Coach Wooten of UCLA said that "Failure is not fatal, but the idea of not changing may be."[1] Place, at a considerable distance behind you, any times of failure—but let those times also teach you and show you a better way to succeed.

Whenever possible, previous successes should be pointed out by the caregiver. In this case, that's me, if you didn't already catch onto that. Noticing periodic successes will only happen if you continuously review where you are against where you have been, and where you want to be. This process will be made easier if you read and reread the parts of this book that pertain specifically to you.

Bertrand Russell, a renowned British philosopher, mathematician, historian, and political activist born in 1872, listed the three passions that governed his life: The longings for love, the search for knowledge, and unbearable pity for the suffering of humankind. The unnecessary suffering of humankind is the passion in my own life that prompted me to write this book. The key word in the sentence is *unnecessary*. My heart goes out to the patients I have worked with who, in spite of my efforts and their efforts, have continued to go down the perilous road of poor lifestyle existence. How to change this is the question of the century.

I've tried to construct the information in this book around five areas of focus:

1. **Identify strengths.** Everyone has strengths. You're having executed the option to read this book already speaks well about your will to do something important and meaningful in your life. That's certainly a strength.
2. **Identify risks.** I will do a great deal of this throughout this book!
3. **Present evidence-based medical information on consequences of unhealthy lifestyle.** We will be knee-deep in that, as well.
4. **Describe the "mismatch"** between where you are and where you should be.
5. **Discuss therapeutic lifestyle changes** and make recommendations that will occur at almost every turn of the page.

What I expect from you, as the reader, is to accept your role as the active partner, embracing the evaluation and proposed treatments throughout this book. Understand from the outset that the program that you will become involved in will not be casual or occasional. Improving your health is a fulltime commitment, and more importantly, a lifelong commitment.

H.P. Blavatsky is the author of this sound, thoughtful bit of philosophy:

---

[1] http://sports.espn.go.com/ncb/news/story?id=5249709

*There is a road, steep and thorny, beset with perils of every kind— but yet a road; and it leads to the heart of the universe. I can tell you how to find those who will show you the secret gateway that leads inward only, and closes fast behind the neophyte for evermore. There is no danger that dauntless courage cannot conquer. There is no trial that spotless purity cannot pass through. There is no difficulty that strong intellect cannot surmount. For those who win onwards, there is reward past all telling: the power to bless and save humanity. For those who fail, there are other lives in which success may come.[2]*

BOTTOM LINE: Write a brief biography about your health, where you are now, and your goals—in other words, the reasons you are reading this book.

---

[2] http://www.universaltheosophy.com/pdf-library/The%20Real%20H.P.%20Blavatsky.pdf

# INTRODUCTION

Why another book on health? There is a great deal of information already out there, and a lot of good stuff, at that. In part, at least, this book was written because of all the information out there—in bookstores, on the Internet, at book kiosks, on the radio and TV. I have seen, read, and listened to it all, and I have filtered the good from the not-so-good. I have sifted through the lukewarm, the misleading, and the often well-meaning medical storehouse of knowledge. And hopefully, I have applied my 53 years of experience in family practice to add validity to my observations and recommendations. After reading this book, you will be equipped to pursue your crusade for better health and a better life.

What this book is not: With a rare exception, it is not a book of anecdotal stories about patients who had horrible lab stats but found religion and turned their illnesses into a sensational health profiles. Rather than someone else's story, this is going to be *your* story. A story you can tell your family and friends when you turn your life around.

At the end of the preface, I suggested writing down a very brief biography briefly—maybe 500 words or less about where you are now. Somewhere down the line, probably months from now, you'll rewrite this biography and reassess your goals and any transformations you've achieved. Deal? Deal!

Do you want to change? I'm guessing, if you are reading this book, that the answer is "yes."

Colin Campbell, author of *The China Study,* said, "There is no greater disrespect a doctor can show patients than that of withholding potentially lifesaving information based on the assumption that patients do not want to change their lifestyle." I will give you all of the lifesaving information you can digest. So don't come to the fire hydrant of this book with only a thimble; you're going to need a big bucket. In fact, you may learn more than you really want to know.

However, using all the information I give you to actually impact your life will take some work. Status quo, "the existing state of affairs," is a very, very powerful force. Most of America is comfortable in "the existing state of affairs." The easiest thing in the world to do is to play it safe and maintain the status quo. The outcomes of new decisions are fraught with uncertainty, and errors can be costly, so sticking with what worked in the past often seems like a safe option, as long as our previous decisions were "good enough."

Abandoning the status quo means making difficult choices and acting on them. Sometimes, it may seem in our best interests to simply do nothing and just maintain our current course. Psychologists tell us that the status quo holds within it the assumption of the longevity and goodness of a position. People simply assume, with little reason or deliberation, the goodness of their existing state—the status quo. Even though choosing the status quo may entail forfeiting positive consequences, the potential gains are often given less weight than the losses that would be incurred if the status quo were changed.

We fear that we will regret making a wrong decision. This is called "loss aversion"—when one is more concerned about losses that may occur when moving away from the status quo than with what may be gained. A tendency to overemphasize the avoidance of losses will thus favor retaining the status quo, resulting in a status quo bias.

Change, then, is put off altogether, and a potential "mover and shaker" will instead stick with what has always been done in the past. The enemy to abandoning the status quo is inertia. It takes more than we presently have in us to get of off dead center.

If your status quo is being sedentary, ignoring healthy eating habits, and carrying around excess body fat, the reality is that there is little goodness in your present status quo. Are you happy right now with "good enough"? A change from the status quo will typically involve both gains and losses. The change will have good overall consequences if the gains outweigh the losses.

As you read this book, I hope you will be convinced that the information you will be harvesting will make your decision to pursue optimal lifestyle change the right decision.

A personal note: I have had good health and I have needed very little medical care throughout my life. Rarely have I been on the other end of the stethoscope. That's a good thing, but it does have its drawbacks. I began practicing in July of 1960 and retired in August of 2013. In all that length of time, I missed only three days of work when I was diagnosed with German measles, and missed one day after sustaining five fractured ribs in a bicycle accident. The downside of this is that I didn't have much experience as a patient.

But as a caregiver for a first wife who died of acute myeloid leukemia and a second wife with a severe lung infection, I have often found myself in waiting rooms, emergency departments, doctor offices, infusion centers, and radiology waiting rooms. Because of this, I now better understand what it means to have compassionate, skilled, and understanding caregivers. I have witnessed doctors, nurses, and even housekeeping personnel extend tenderness and encouragement to my loved ones. I am grateful for their services. I will note one exception—a seven-and-a-half-hour emergency room visit that could have been much, much shorter. But they're working on it, and when I left a note, the administrator did get back to me, saying, "Thanks for your note, and for your feedback. I apologize to you and your wife for the long wait and for the inefficiencies in our processes of care. It is something we are constantly working on and certainly can continue to improve." Such is the challenge of a busy emergency room.

Let me relate one of the most noteworthy sports stories on record, about a surprising hero who once played with Mickey Mantle and Yogi Berra. He was a right-hander, and on one extraordinary day, October 8, 1956, with 64,519 people watching, he retired 27 batters without giving up one hit. This no-hitter was the Yankees vs. the Brooklyn Dodgers in a 1956 World Series game.

The rest of his 14-year career, spent with eight different teams, consisted of mediocrity interspersed with moments of competence. He never led his league in any category. To his credit, his World Series record was 4 to 2 with a 2.75 ERA. As a hitter, he had a lifetime batting average of .242 with 14 homers. That is pretty good for a pitcher.

Who was this unusual man who spun a no-hitter in the fifth game of the 1956 World Series? It wasn't Don Drysdale or Sandy Koufax. His name was Don Larsen. In the 1965 season, Larsen was traded to the Orioles, for whom he went 1 for 2. He concluded his career in 1967, pitching three games for the Cubs. After spending 1966 and most of the next season in the minors, he pitched three games for the Cubs at the tail end of 1967. Larsen retired after 14 seasons with a record of 81 to 91.

The point of this story is that Don Larsen had a no-hitter in him, and he got the opportunity to put into play that singular accomplishment. I know you have a no-hitter in you, too. Pitch one for the Old Gipper, but better still, pitch one for yourself and those you love and those who want you around for a long, long time. With this book, you will now have the "home team advantage" in the contact sport that is life.

BOTTOM LINE: If you haven't already, write a brief autobiography. Then write down how you are willing to change.

*Note: I've learned a lot of facts and statistics over my decades in family practice, and I did not always write down where I got them from. Although many of these facts are simply entrenched in my mind, whenever possible, I will reference sources for any factual information I impart to you. I will also recommend resources for further reading about some topics.*

# SOMETHING'S NOT RIGHT!

Two cavemen are talking to one another: "Something's not right. Our air is clean, our water is pure, we all get plenty of exercise, everything we eat is organic and free-range, and yet nobody lives past 30." That is a perplexing pronouncement. If you will be patient and work through the chapters in this book, I will explain the mismatch.

In this one big enormous world, under the same sun, moon, and stars, how can we all breath the same polluted air and yet be so different, health-wise? Rates of cancer in various parts of the world differ enormously. Twenty-some years ago, China exhibited a rarity of heart disease, versus the United States' staggering rate. That has changed as China has embraced the Western ways of self-destruction by abandoning their dietary ideals. There have been relatively swift changes in disease, which cannot be assigned to genetic differences between populations. Instead, they are due to differences in lifestyle, with dietary factors and physical activity being the causative factors.

To be so bold as to state that good health depends upon diet and exercise could be offensive to those whose lifestyle, day in and day out, is to simply default to denying what is good for them. To report that attention to correct and scientifically proven lifestyles improves mortality rates is an important motivation for maintaining a healthful lifestyle. Mortality is something we are all concerned about, but morbidity is at least as important—quality of life matters.

Sixty to seventy-five percent of first coronary events are not fatal, but can lead to great economic burden and substantial premature disability. We shouldn't overlook the dramatic adverse health changes a non-fatal coronary event can bring about on the general quality of life, causing other nonfatal conditions such as cognitive decline to memory and thought process. To only view death rates and the accompanying statistics in our analysis of our cultural health would be an undersight. "You are either dead or you're not" is a fallacy, or at least, the full impact of being one or the other is not appreciated. I don't want my own end-of-life bonus to be just one week less in I.C.U. or two months shorter in the nursing home. I want to be active and contributing to my family and community until my birth certificate expires.

It is there for us to use, but we have to believe in it, grab the golden ring, and move forward. I'm talking about the myriad of evidence that tells us how to be healthier and happier, and contribute more to family, community, and self. Without resolve, however, that data and evidence are meaningless.

## Who Is In Charge of Your Health?

Who really is in charge of your health? More importantly, who is going to see that your life can be of the quality that you deserve? There are three possibilities: the government, the team, and YOU. Lets take a good look at these three options.

**Government:** The authors of the book *Habits in the Heart: Individualism and Commitment in American Life* advance the ideas that:

> *Our problems are individual or in only a narrow sense social (that is, involving family and local community), rather than economic, political, and cultural. A related feature that these common explanations of our troubles share is hostility to the role of government or the state. If we can take care of ourselves, perhaps with a little help from our friends and family, who needs the state? Indeed, the state is often viewed as an interfering father who won't recognize that his children have grown up and don't need him anymore. He can't help solve our problems because it is in large measure he who created them."* [3]

These are some good points, which set up the background for my feelings about "an interfering father." Admittedly, the government is faced with some big challenges, and with medical care being 17.9 percent of the Gross Domestic Product (GDP)[4] in 2012 compared to 2 percent in 1970[5], medical care is way up there as a cost of living expense.

The current Congress and administration seem unable—or, probably more accurately, unwilling—to face the biggest challenge in medicine, the cost of medical care. The Affordable Care Act ("Obamacare") does have its problems, among which is the actual cost of the program. The government currently does little to cut down on medical expenditures, but eventually it will have to. When it comes to cutting corners, reducing reimbursement to physicians looks pretty good to our government, but obviously less attractive to physicians, and reimbursement cuts have already taken place.

Lets look at this more closely and see if it will impact your medical care.

In a May 2008 issue, *The Journal of the American Medical Association (JAMA)* reported:

> *The Affordable Care Act will also reduce physician reimbursement.*

---

[3] *Habits of the Heart, Individualism and Commitment in American Life*, Robert N. Bellah, Richard Madsen, William M. Sullivan, Ann Swidler, Steven M. Tipton http://www.ucpress.edu/book.php?isbn=9780520254190
[4] World Bank Data http://data.worldbank.org/indicator/SH.XPD.TOTL.ZS
[5] USGovernmentSpending.com: http://www.usgovernmentspending.com/healthcare_spending

*The Affordable Care Act's decreases will undermine patient's access to care. There is currently a shortage of physicians, especially primary care physicians. Reimbursement cuts will compound the problem by discouraging physicians from treating Medicare and Medicaid patients and potentially discouraging students from becoming physicians. Many physicians have already refused to accept Medicare payments because of low fees that have markedly declined over the past 20 years.[6]*

If the Affordable Care Act achieves one of its goals, more patients may have insurance, but will doctors welcome them into their practices? Fees will be discounted, the cost of doing business as a physician will continue to go up, and doctors may be forced to reconsider taking on certain patients.

I spoke of the cost of medicine. James Heskett, a Baker Foundation Professor, Emeritus, at Harvard Business School, has this to say, "To put things in perspective, U.S. healthcare currently costs about $2 trillion per year. Of this, more than $600 billion (31 percent) is never seen by recipients. It goes for administration." In the private sector, the administrative cost is closer to 20 percent. Heskett continues, "On a per capita basis, it is roughly $280 billion more than is spent for administration in the other twenty-one countries whose life expectancies exceed those in the U.S."[7] You might want to re-read that statement.

**Medicare/Medicaid:** The government is borrowing from social security to pay for Medicare, essentially writing an I.O.U to itself. Statistics from 2012 show that Medicare spending, which represents 20 percent of national health spending, costs $572.5 billion. Medicaid, accounting for 14.7 percent, registers $421.2 billion.[8] Both of these will increase yearly as more and more people get older and into Medicare. Obamacare throws a widening net and will include more people than are now covered on Medicaid, so simple mathematics tells us there will be greater costs in this arena.

In the U.S., each person's financial exposure (liability) and what we actually owe in debt amounts to an average of $150,000 per person. But if you distribute that over the fulltime work force, it averages around $370,000 per fulltime worker, according to 2011 figures.[9] In the U.S., we spend $8,915 per person on healthcare.[10] Norway, the Netherlands, and Switzerland are the next

---

[6] The Journal of the American Medical Association
http://jama.jamanetwork.com/issues.aspx?journalID=67&year=2009#issues_tabContentWrapper

[7] Harvard Business School's Working Knowledge newsletter, "What Is the Government's Role in U.S. Healthcare?" March 2, 2007 http://hbswk.hbs.edu/item/5645.html

[8] http://www.cms.gov/Research-Statistics-Data-and-Systems/Statistics-Trends-and-Reports/NationalHealthExpendData/NHE-Fact-Sheet.html

[9] Dr. Brent James, BYU Forum, March 18, 2014

[10] http://www.cms.gov/Research-Statistics-Data-and-Systems/Statistics-Trends-and-Reports/NationalHealthExpendData/NationalHealthAccountsHistorical.html

highest spenders, but in the same year, they all spent at least $3,000 less per person.[11] The average spending on healthcare among the other 33 developed OECD countries was $3,268 per person.[12] We rank below 16 other rich countries in the world with our healthcare results, and results are a very important part of what really counts! Relatively speaking, we aren't doing that well.

Most of those in Congress believe the financial crisis will come after they leave their government posts. They see their job as simply to get elected now, and cutting down on spending and entitlements will make re-election less likely. This is how the system functions. The government has power and is likely to continue to use it, but it will probably come in the form of rationing, in that treatment for certain diseases, specific procedures, and the specific ages of those being treated will be determined by the government—someone sitting at a desk with a computer in front of them—not the patient. Graphs and charts will be used to determine who gets what—not individual considerations, something we now enjoy to some extent. The government "fix-it programs" have a poor track record in healthcare, so don't depend on government to meet your healthcare needs. As far as I have noticed, they have a poor track record on most economic policies.

The government seems to have its hands not only in our pocketbooks, but also in our grocery baskets. The U.S. Department of Agriculture (USDA) is the proponent and voice of our food industry. Every five years, the USDA comes out with updated nutritional guidelines for the public. These guidelines are primarily driven by profit from food sales; the USDA is not overly concerned with the health advantages or disadvantages of the foods they recommend. But with the right, proven recommendations, you should be able to sort through this often subjective advice.

**The Team:** Who is "the team?" It includes all sorts of people in medical offices, clinics, and hospitals. My intention is not to destroy your trust in medical caregivers, for they have a huge challenge in delivering medical care, particularly in this day and age. Most of the time, we medical caregivers make the right decisions, but because of our human limitations, we don't always come up with the right answers.

Professor Sir Cyril Chantler, the first Chair of UCL Partners, Europe's largest academic health science partnership, said, "Medicine used to be simple, ineffective, and relatively safe. Now it is complex, effective, and potentially dangerous."[13] Some of the challenges seem almost too difficult to overcome. For example, keeping up with medical knowledge and skill is a real challenge. Medical research and knowledge proliferates rapidly.

---

11 http://www.pbs.org/newshour/rundown/health-costs-how-the-us-compares-with-other-countries/

12 http://www.oecd.org/health/health-systems/49084355.pdf

13 "The role and education of doctors in the delivery of healthcare," *Chantler C Lancet. 1999 Apr 3; 353(9159):1178-81.*

Before modern medicine, doctors held hands, named diseases, and predicted outcomes. Now, a whole lot more occurs. Doctors change the course of lives, for the better. They help improve the quality of lives, as well as extending years to the lives of many people. But this only occurs as patients internalize accurate and effective information about optimal lifestyle.

The U.S. healthcare system is characterized by information overload. There is more to know, more to do, and more to manage and correlate than at any other time in history. This has resulted in extraordinary complexity. "Medicare patients now see an average of seven physicians, including five specialists, split among four different practices, for their healthcare. In a single year, a typical primary care physician coordinates with an average of 229 other physicians in 117 different practices just for that physician's Medicare patient population."[14]

MEDLINE, the National Library of Medicine for database collection, draws citations from approximately 5,600 worldwide journals in 39 languages. About 45 percent come from cited articles published in the U.S. Since 2005, between 2,000 to 4,000 completed references have been added four days a week, every week—there were nearly 700,000 added in 2010 alone. The majority of the publications covered in MEDLINE are scholarly journals; a small number of newspapers, magazines, and newsletters are also considered useful.

With all of this information, it is rather obvious that a physician couldn't possibly have the access, the time, or the inclination to read even a small part of this vast storehouse of medical knowledge. To stay thoroughly up-to-date, a primary care physician would need to read twenty papers a day, 365 days of the year—an impossible task. Over 2,500 clinical practice guidelines pervade medical practice. Guidelines are constructed to afford the physician evidence-based information to better direct the care of a particular patient. Again, a daunting task to keep up with.

Is this information always applicable, and will it continue to be useful? Today's truth may be tomorrow's folly. The half-life of truth in medicine is short. There is an axiom in medicine: "Half of what is true today will be proven to be incorrect in the next five years. Unfortunately, we don't know which half that is going to be."[15] That is how fast knowledge is being discovered.

I have heard Dr. Brent James of the Intermountain Healthcare System, based in Salt Lake City, state, "An internist three to four years out of residency and board certification begins to show significant declines in general medical knowledge."

I would now like to quote Dr. Lawrence Weed, a longtime professor at the University of Vermont. Dr. Weed had much to do with the "problem-oriented medical record" (POMR) so extensively used by the medical community for record-keeping.

---

[14] New England Journal of Medicine 2007; 12 (2):143-147

[15] Lakshmipati G. Care of the medical outpatient, (Preface) 1st ed. 2003. pp. vii–vii. Nama publication, Coimbatore, Tamilnadu.

*Only a portion of medical knowledge is ever loaded into the minds of professionals. Not all of the knowledge loaded in the minds of professionals is retained, and much of the knowledge that professionals retain becomes obsolete, and there is no assurance that they will learn new knowledge relevant to their patients' problems. Even with the limited knowledge that it retains, a doctor's unaided mind cannot reliably integrate that knowledge with the infinite variety of data about patients in order to identify and systematically assess all diagnostic or treatment options based on each patient's unique characteristics and needs.[16]*

There is not a doctor who doesn't face these challenges, by the way. Even the "super specialist" whose whole life's work is operating on the right knee faces the issue of knowing everything there is to know about that right knee.

Enter the computer. We notice, as we sit down in the doctor's examining room, that she is facing the computer, and often not looking at the patient. After all, the computer is where all the information and answers to your health questions are—or at least you would think. You also undoubtedly notice that there now is limited eye contact and lack of touching. The science of medicine is the computer, but the art of medicine is touching. So, we have lost the art of medicine to the better of two virtues, science. I leave this statement for you to think about.

Without the computer, we could not comply with the government's attempt to make the entire nation dependent upon electronic health records. We no longer have paperwork, just computer work. Sounds good to healthcare professionals, and probably is good, to some extent. But does it provide the high quality healthcare we as physicians so earnestly desire?

According to a study by the RAND Corporation in late 2013, physicians in general say the systems are cumbersome and are a significant contributor to job dissatisfaction. Those who were surveyed felt there was too much time spent performing clerical work, and that it encouraged template-generated notes, thus depersonalizing one-on-one contact with the patient, in addition to providing inaccurate information designed to cover everyone with the same blanket.

Four years ago, I decided to become a "shadow" in specialists' offices. I would call the caregiver, present my case, and ask for a half-day in their presence. Being a "shadow" means sitting quietly in the same room as the specialist and his patient and observing, without commenting on what the visit was all about and how the doctor and patient came to the diagnosis and treatment. This was an experience that I treasured. I learned things about medicine and doctors that you don't find in books or at the feet of the lecturing medical expert. Being a compulsive person, I wrote down the whole experience,

---

16

http://www.bmj.com/lookup/ijlink?linkType=FULL&journalCode=bmj&resid=315/7102/231&atom=%2Fbmj%2F321%2F7265%2F878.atom

noting the medical knowledge that I encountered and any other revelations that occurred.

In this experience with 26 different caregivers, including psychiatrists, chiropractors, and physical therapists, I came away with a couple of things which spoke more of the culture that is being created with the doctor-patient encounter perhaps than any esoteric treatment modality. I noticed very little touching of patients (especially at the nephrologist's office), but I came away with an increased respect for my colleagues regarding the administration of their skills and knowledge. Their style may have been different than mine, but I appreciated their integrity as they attempted to solve patients' health challenges and reassure their patients about their health.

Please don't get me wrong about the medical community. It is the best we've got, and we are trying harder and harder to deliver good medical care. But there are inherent problems in medicine. In the December 18, 2013 issue of *Journal of the American Medical Association*, we get some pretty startling figures:

> *Preventable harm is the third leading cause of patient death, and one-third of healthcare spending—estimated at nearly $1 trillion, or $9000 per household—is for therapies that do not improve patients' health. One estimate suggests that each year, 200 000 patients die from sepsis (infection), 120,000 from teamwork failures, 100,000 from healthcare–acquired infections, 100,000 from venous thromboembolism and pulmonary embolus (clots to the lungs), 80,000 from diagnostic errors, and 68,000 from decubitus ulcers.*[17]

We can't insure patients will live forever. The preventable harm scenario is not necessarily default on the part of caregivers, but the natural history of health and disease plays a major role in what may be taken as inadequacy and neglect in the healthcare system.

*The American Medical News* of January 28, 2013 tells us that 50 million operations are done each year in the U.S. There is one adverse "event that never should have happened" in 12,248 procedures.[18] About the failure to follow procedures and use checklists that would prevent such issues, Dr. Dagi, a neurosurgeon, said "It's got to be done right everywhere. Patients have a right to it, and it's our responsibility to see that right is protected."[19] The majority of these errors are the results of surgical instruments (such as sponges) unintentionally left behind in patients, entirely wrong procedures being performed, and procedures being performed on the wrong surgical site. Researchers found

---

[17] http://jama.jamanetwork.com/issue.aspx?journalid=67&issueid=929490

[18]

http://www.pwrnewmedia.com/2013/joint_commission/big_news_january/download_cth/cth_surgical_errors_-in_or.pdf

[19] http://www.amednews.com/article/20130121/profession/130129976/2/

nearly 10,000 cases of these types of errors, totaling $1.3 billion in legal settlements, over a 20-year period.[20]

**YOU:** Now we are getting down to the real business of my message to you! This is an ever-changing world. In 2000,125 million people were affected by chronic conditions. The estimates are that by 2020 this will increase to about 157 million[21]. There are increasing numbers of YOUs.

What is this all about, and what am I really building a case for? YOU have stuck it out this long… now comes the answer to *who is really in charge of your healthcare.* Unequivocally it is YOU. In my practice, I always tried to get my patients to take responsibility for their own health, because YOU are the most cost effective of the three possibilities, YOU are the most likely to succeed, and YOU will produce the greatest positive outcome. Now that is worth a great deal.

After reading this book you should be able to incorporate the information I will give you into your plan, and then success will be yours, whether it be to lose weight, become physically stronger, have more vitality, or formulate and stick to a healthy exercise program. Don't let this scare you, but the onus is directly on YOU. "If it's going to be it's up to me." That has been my motto most of my life. Now let it be yours!

My role is to identify risks as described on the written page, present evidence-based medical information on the consequences of an unhealthy lifestyle, and point out the mismatch between where you are and where you should be. Then I will offer you a number of choices—some better than others, but most healthier than your present lifestyle. We will then become partners in the most impactful undertaking of your whole life.

BOTTOM LINE: Healthcare rationing is an eventuality. Doctors do all they can, but are not perfect. YOU are in charge of your future, and that is exactly who should be in charge.

---

[20] http://www.amednews.com/article/20130121/profession/130129976/2/

[21] http://www.amga.org/wcm/PI/Collabs/MPMCC/index_mpmcc.aspx

# CURRENT HEALTH STANDINGS

I would like to see us all at our optimal health. As long as we are making goals and putting our efforts into this area of our lives, let's shoot for the best. According to the World Health Organization, *optimal health* is defined as "a state of optimal well-being, not merely the absence of disease and infirmity."[22] Keep this premise in mind as we move forward.

Is our lifestyle really so bad that there is no hope? Our lifestyle might be bad, but there is always hope.

In order to give you a sense of where the United States is with our present state of health, and the enormous hill we need to climb to be where we ought to be, I am about to give you a lot of information. If statistics don't interest you, I give you permission to go to the BOTTOM LINE at the end of this chapter for the simple summary.

Anyone can make a point by manipulating statistics. Take, for example, the story of the freshman in college, away from home and family for the first time. To please his father, he went out for track. He had no athletic ability, though the father had been a good miler in his day. The freshman's first race was a two-man race in which he ran against the school miler. He was badly beaten. Not wanting to disappoint his father, the boy wrote home as follows: "You will be happy to know that I ran against Bill Hansen, the best miler in school. He came in next-to-last, while I came in second."

Data from large population studies suggests that lifestyle factors, such as a sedentary habit, dietary intake, and obesity, are responsible for up to 70 percent of chronic diseases and are a major contributor to reduced longevity.

The graph below compares the year 2010 to the year 1990 and gives life expectancy and healthy life expectancy figures.

| Years | Life expectancy | Healthy Life expectancy |
|---|---|---|
| 1990 | 75.2 years | 65.8 |
| 2010 | 78.2 years | 68.1 |
| Change in years | 3 | 2.3 |

Life expectancy is the expected number of years of life remaining at a given age. We most often calculate life expectancy from birth. Because life expectancy is an average, a particular person may die many years before or many years after his "expected" survival age. U.S. life expectancy overall increased from 75.2 years in 1990 to 78.2 years in 2010; during the same period,

---

[22] http://www.livestrong.com/article/277873-the-definition-of-optimal-health/

healthy life expectancy (HALE) increased from 65.8 years to 68.1 years. HALE refers to years of productivity and good health—not merely being alive.[23]

The point is, your healthy life expectancy is, as of 2010 figures, is 10.1 years shorter than your total life expectancy. To me, that speaks to quality of life, or, better said, the less-than-optimal quality of end of life.

Fifty percent of adults have one or more chronic diseases. The diseases that we can do most about are heart disease, obesity, diabetes, high blood pressure, and cancer. Just a few statistics and comments about each:

**Heart Disease:** About 600,000 people die of heart disease in the United States every year—one in every four deaths. Each year, about 720,000 Americans have a heart attack.[24] Seventy-one million Americans (33.5 percent) have "bad cholesterol."[25] Less than half are treated for it. People with bad cholesterol have twice the risk of heart disease than those with optimal levels.

**Obesity:** A whopping 35.1 percent of Americans are obese, and 69 percent are considered overweight or obese based on BMI (body mass index) standards.[26] There is hardly a disease that is not worsened by obesity. The Quality Improvement Initiative showed every extra 10 pounds of body weight shortens the period before the onset of heart disease by a year and a half; the average American is nearly 30 pounds overweight. White men from 20 to 30 with a severe level of obesity can expect a shorter life by 13 years, and white women, 8 years.[27] For men, this could represent a 22 percent reduction in their expected remaining life span.

**Diabetes:** In the U.S., 9.3 percent of the population suffers from diabetes. An additional 86 million adults are considered to be pre-diabetic. In those 65 years and older, the rate of diabetes is 25.9 percent.[28] Diabetes is the leading cause of kidney failure, non-traumatic lower limb amputation, and new blindness in adults. Diabetes is also a major cause of strokes and heart attacks. Seventy percent of diabetics will die of a heart attack.

**High Blood Pressure:** Sixty-seven million American adults (31 percent) have high blood pressure—one in three. Fifty-three percent do not adequately control it. One in three American adults has prehypertension. There are 1,000

---

[23] The State of U.S. Health, 1990-2010, Burden of Disease, injuries, & Risk Factors, JAMA July10, 2013 Pg 591

[24] http://www.cdc.gov/heartdisease/facts.htm

[25] http://www.cdc.gov/cholesterol/facts.htm

[26] http://www.cdc.gov/nchs/fastats/obesity-overweight.htm

[27] *Years of Life Are Lost Due to Obesity,* Reprinted from *Eating Disorders Review,* May/June 2003 Volume 14, Number 3 ©2003 Gürze Books

[28] http://www.diabetes.org/diabetes-basics/statistics/

deaths daily from high blood pressure.[29] High blood pressure puts a person at risk for heart attacks, heart failure, and strokes.

**Cancer:** Cancer claims more than half a million lives per year.[30] Many in the field of preventive medicine suggest that 30 to 40 percent of all cancers are related to unhealthy eating habits.[31] Medical experts unanimously agree that all five chronic diseases are linked to the modern Western diet. However, they disagree on how to prevent or cure them. Within this book, I believe I can clarify some of the questions and inconsistencies on how one should approach these diseases.

But first, how does our marvelous "head of the pack" country compare with the rest of the world?

Among the 34 countries studied between 1990 and 2010, here is the U.S. ranking.[32]

| HALE (healthy life expectancy) | Fell from 14th to 26th |
|---|---|
| YLLs (years of life lost to premature mortality) | Fell from 23rd to 28th |
| YLDs (years lived with disability) | Fell from 5th to 6th |

Again, when we're talking about HALE figures, "healthy life expectancy" refers to the average number of years that a newborn can expect to live in full health. The expression "full health" implies continued productivity and enjoyment of life. HALE tries to measure a health system's effectiveness in reducing the burden of illness. Sometimes, an illness can be shortened or suffering reduced, yet the mortality rate doesn't change. HALE was established to assess the health system's ability to reduce suffering *even if the mortality rate remains unchanged.* HALE is a calculation used by statisticians and demographers to adjust life expectancy for the amount of time spent in poor health. Pretty tedious, isn't it! I encourage you to keep reading, and am certainly not expecting you to remember all the figures.

Below, I have selected several countries to give a perspective of where we in the United States fit within world HALE numbers.

| | |
|---|---|
| Japan | 75 |
| Switzerland | 73 |
| Canada | 72 |
| United Kingdom | 72 |

---

[29] http://www.cdc.gov/bloodpressure/facts.htm

[30] http://www.cancer.org/research/cancerfactsstatistics/cancerfactsfigures2014/index

[31] http://www.breastcancer.org/risk/factors/unhealthy_food

[32] The State of U.S. Health, 1990-2010, JAMA July 2013

| Iceland | 70 |
| United States | 69 |
| Cuba | 68 |
| Mexico | 65 |
| China | 64 |
| Brazil | 60 |
| Pakistan | 53 |
| Haiti | 44 |
| Liberia | 35 |

These numbers were calculated by taking into account years lived in less than full health due to disease and/or injury. I did not include all of the countries that do a better job than we do. The U.S. HALE, according to a 2013 report, went from 14th to 26th. That is not what we want to see. We have obviously done very poorly keeping up our quality of life. The average U.S. male can expect to live almost four fewer years than men in the top-ranked countries. This trend is concerning!

In a study of 2,390 people, many patients who had conventional risk factors for coronary heart disease achieved goal levels without medications within 12 weeks of initiating therapeutic lifestyle changes.[33] This finding refutes the notion that intensive lifestyle intervention is not worth the effort. Just think, there is a way out of this mess—not an easy way, but a proven way.

## The Cost of Our Indiscretions

| | | |
|---|---|---|
| 2012 | According to the World Health Organization (WHO), the United States spent on healthcare per capita | $8,608 |
| 1993 | healthcare cost per person/year | $3,000 |
| 2011 | average family healthcare cost/year | $19,393 |
| 2021 | average family healthcare cost/year | $42,000 |
| 1970 | GDP (gross domestic product) for medical care | 7% |
| 2012 | GDP for medical care. | 16%[34] |

The U.S. spends more per capita on healthcare than any other nation, yet is ranked last in the quality of healthcare among similar countries. Every year, according to the 2012 Milliman Medical Index, every U.S. family of four pays the dollar equivalent of a new Chevy Cruze in healthcare costs.

---

[33] http://www.hypnotension.com/news/how-to-lower-your-blood-pressure-in-12-weeks-without-drugs/
[34] http://www.who.int/en/

| DATE | CONSUMED BY EACH PERSON EACH YEAR[35] |
|---|---|
| Turn of the 20th Century | 120 pounds of meat |
| 2007 | 222 pounds of meat |
| 1913 | 40 pounds of processed sugar |
| 2012 | 82 pounds of processed sugar |
| 1909 | 294 pounds of dairy products |
| 2006 | 605 pounds of dairy products |
| Currently | 41.5 pounds of high-fructose corn syrup |
| Currently | 65 pounds fat (2 tons suet by age 60) |

We now each consume 41.5 pounds of fructose, via corn syrup, a year,[36] and that is not good. From 1909-2004, per capita cheese intake rose from less than 4 pounds per year to nearly 34 pounds.[37] (Cheese is rich in saturated fat. More later about that.)

Another way to look at America's health status is to look at our older population. As reported in the *Annals of Long-Term Care*, October 2013, eighty percent of people over the age of 65 have at east one chronic condition, with an average of four per person; this same group uses between two to six prescribed medications and one to three-point-four non-prescribed medications on a regular basis.[38] The National Center for Health Statistics reports that 37 percent of people age 60 and older took five or more different medications, and 76 percent in this age group took two or more different medications.[39]

Even if you're young now, your likelihood of reaching 65 is pretty good. Someday you will become a statistic, if you are not one already. The ultimate in dysfunctional living is dying. Be committed, unwavering, and dedicated to your goals. Be passionate.

At this stage, I would like to suggest that you remove from your lexicon the phrase "just this once." "Just this once" is poison to any program that you are trying to follow. As an example, you are offered a donut at work and you say: "Just this once; after all, I have lost weight these last few days, I am on target, so 'just this once' can't be all that bad." No, no don't eat it!

Or, you decide to sleep in "just this once" and forgo your two-mile morning walk. It seems harmless, but that is marginal thinking. In my experience, "just this once" is a sure path to failure as you try to reach a hard-to-achieve goal. It is easier to maintain your commitment 100 percent of the time than 98 percent of that time. Your actions are hardwired in your brain. You have worked so hard to develop the right kinds of habits, and you must remember that your behavior is

---

[35] http://veggiesforme.com/2011/09/14/shocking-rate-of-increase-of-consumption-of-meat-dairy-and-sugar/

[36] http://institutefornaturalhealing.com/2011/04/a-sweet-death-the-truth-about-high-fructose-corn-syrup/

[37] http://www.cnpp.usda.gov/publications/foodsupply/foodsupply1909-2004report.pdf

[38] http://www.annalsoflongtermcare.com/archive

[39] http://www.cdc.gov/nchs/

on autopilot. Forming good habits and sticking to them is key in your approach to being effective and reaching your goal.

BOTTOM LINE: As individuals and as a country we are doing poorly with our quality of life and longevity. Our major stumbling blocks are sedentary lifestyle and poor dietary habits. We don't have to immediately go to medications. Many patients who have conventional risk factors for coronary heart disease can achieve goal levels without medications within 12 weeks of initiating therapeutic lifestyle changes and refute the notion that intensive lifestyle intervention is not worth the effort. Make a major effort to reduce or eliminate added sugar, meat, and dairy products, including cheese.

# GETTING STARTED

Let's be clear about one of the most important desires in life: optimal health. This is what the various chapters in the book are all about. There are many rewards for optimal health. For some, it may be being able to go higher when "leaping tall buildings in a single bound." For others, it may be being able to get rid of the walker and get to the grocery store unassisted. Right this minute, the possibilities for your obtaining optimal health depend on your age; existing diseases or lack thereof; resources, including social networks; genetics; finances; and so forth. As we were not all created equal, we do not all have the same opportunities, capacity, and resources to be physiologically where we dream to be.

One thing I can promise you is that after reading and studying this book, your definition of optimal health will be at a higher level than you now understand it to be. To quote Napoleon Hill, "A goal is a dream with a deadline." You must become specific around things like:

- Where do I want to be with activity and exercise?
- How much weight do I want to lose?
- How do I change my dietary habits to maximize the nutritional value of what I eat?

To answer these questions will require changes in your lifestyle. I've already asked you to write out your plan and goals, and also to write about where you are and where you want to be. I hope you have done so.

Where does one find the power to become successful in the quest for good health and happiness? Where does one find the power, if you will, to actually make changes in her life? Maybe "power" isn't the right word, or maybe other descriptors would be better—like, say motivation. You must have something secure in your life, such as a belief in yourself. Believing in yourself must be the cornerstone of faith in what you are doing. Be patient with your struggles and the direction you should take, and trust in the integrity you are showing to begin the process of change. Integrity, to me, is how close your performance is to what your principles and guiding tenets in life are. Integrity is the bedrock of character. And character is what is left over after the hype is gone. There will undoubtedly be some hype in the subsequent pages of this book. You may have to sift through a little of that to get to the rock-hard foundation. But it is there.

You may be burning the candle at both ends, and attempting to lose weight or exercise may feel just another project and too much to take on at this time. After all, there is a limit; a person can take just so much. You have to decide when too much is too much!

In other words, you have to be able to correctly draw the Plimsoll line in your life. Samuel Plimsoll was a member of the English Parliament in the 1800s. He was distressed because cargo ships were being loaded so heavily that they were sinking at sea, resulting in much loss of life and property. So he got a law passed requiring danger lines to be painted on all cargo ships. When the weight taken on lowered the ship down to where the line touched the water, all loading had to stop. It turned out to be a good law.

Seamen still call this mark *the Plimsoll line*. People, too, have Plimsoll lines. Having been given this caution about "overload," you must realize the value of the cargo you are about to take on. Therapeutic lifestyle change is more valuable than other "baggage" you may be carrying now. You may be able to add on to your present agenda of activity guiding your health goals. But, if you've already reached your personal Plimsoll line, push overboard the less important, inconsequential cargo in lieu of that which has value. Stop trying to gather up things that don't matter. Besides, you can never get enough of those things. Health is what matters!

Be patient with yourself. You will make mistakes. You will have momentary setbacks. Don't let the past ruin your future.

Put away your past failures at weight reduction and not being able to break the late-night routine of ice cream indulgence, or preferring to lay on the couch watching your favorite NBA team lose rather than taking a walk around the block. Know that in spite of your strong resolve you will not always see the immediate reward. All good things take time! You have walked to the waters of the Red Sea before, and they have opened for you at the last minute. They will part for you again.

Success will, in part, be based upon what you can see in the future and how firmly you can grasp the information in this book. As we go along, I will make clear the potential for the future.

BOTTOM LINE: "Life ultimately means taking the responsibility to find the right answer to its problems and to fulfill the tasks which it constantly sets for each individual." — Viktor Frankl

# PERIODIC HEALTH EXAMINATION

Before you begin making any of the lifestyle changes recommended in this book, do you need to contact your physician? Most likely not. If you are sedentary or have coexistent diseases, such as high blood pressure or cholesterol problems, or are just not sure about your present health status, then a visit and an examination may be appropriate.

In that case, should you get just a "regular" exam or should you schedule a complete physical? People often ask me how often they should get a physical or whether they really need one. Let me attempt to elucidate this often confusing dilemma of whether to be seen, examined, evaluated, and counseled when one is "well." Some call it a "physical." Other names are "wellness exam," "periodic health assessment," and "routine check-up." We in the medical community refer to it as a "periodic health evaluation," or PHE. The PHE has been a fundamental part of medical practice for decades, despite a lack of consensus on its value. These types of exams are really a North American phenomenon, and not pervasive in other parts of the world.

The PHE is a visit with a healthcare provider or team to assess your overall health. Most importantly, the PHE is an encounter designed to identify risk factors for preventable disease through history, physical examination, and appropriate lab testing. Based on the information obtained by providers, patients will receive counseling, immunizations, perhaps referrals to specialists, and appropriate follow-up when necessary.

Those who spend their time analyzing outcomes in the medical world find the visit and what is done at that visit heterogeneous, at best. The items in the PHE have a wide variation, often making it difficult to come to clear conclusions about the value of the exam. The specifics of the PHE depend on who is doing the exam, the age of the patient, and why the physical is being done. In adults, PHEs often focus on diet, physical activity, alcohol and substance abuse factors, and smoking risks.

The big question: What is the evidence that a PHE, delivered at different patient ages or different frequencies, is associated with benefits compared to care without a PHE?

Let's go beyond our borders and get an opinion from the Canadian Task Force on Preventative Care (CTF). Established in 1976, the U.S. has long respected their research and longevity in the field of preventable medicine. Long before we got into the game in1979, CTF determined that the undefined "annual checkup" should be abandoned and replaced with a series of age-specific "health protective packages" implemented during the course of medical visits for other purposes.

*The Annals of Internal Medicine* tells us:

*The best available evidence assessing benefits or harms of the PHE consisted of 21 studies published from 1973 to 2004. The PHE had a consistently beneficial association with the patient receiving (for women) a gynecologic examination and a Papanicolaou (Pap) smear, cholesterol screening, and fecal occult blood testing. The PHE also had a beneficial effect on patient "worry" in one randomized, controlled trial but had mixed effects on other clinical outcomes and costs.[40]*

Seems a little unclear in regard to having a strong recommendation for or against the PHE. Note that in 2013, the Society of General Internal Medicine recommended against routine health checks.

Another voice in the PHE wilderness, Allan Goroll, MACP, a professor of medicine at Harvard Medical School and a practicing general internist:

*There's little evidence that a routine physical exam and a standard 20-30 item chemical panel improve outcomes. However, there is substantial evidence that checking for and treating cardiovascular risk factors, preventable or curable cancers, STDs (sexually transmitted diseases), depression and substance abuse are all evidence-based, high-value activities.[41]*

The United States Services Task Force Recommendation tells us we start PHEs too early and perform them too often, for too long; there needs to be a balance between the benefit, risk, and cost. For younger and middle aged adults, less frequent exams seem appropriate—every three to five years. The PHE has mixed effects on costs, disability, hospitalization, and mortality.

How do patients feel about the PHE? According to a study assessing patient feelings and expectations of the PHE, over 90 percent are in favor of the examination on a yearly basis. Additionally, patients want extensive laboratory and other procedures, over and above that which are recommended. I think that our healthcare system and physicians drive this strong advocacy for the PHE in particular.

Recent legislation will provide coverage at no cost for a "Welcome to Medicare Visit" for new enrollees, incorporating a range of diagnoses and screening tests.

Whether we call it a PHE, a physical, or whatever, the patient and doctor need to get together to map out a "rest of your life" health strategy. The exam we have been talking about is a good time to do this; nonetheless, the "bells and whistles" of the PHE can be eliminated so that both physician and patient can receive education and motivation to change the patient's lifestyle, when

---

[40] The Annals of Internal Medicine 2007 Feb 20;146(4):289-300
http://annals.org/issue.aspx?journalid=90&issueid=20131

[41] ACP Internist, January 2010 http://www.acpinternist.org/archives/2010/01/annual.htm

appropriate. This could be done at another time in the physician's schedule, but that must be determined by the physician and his style of delivering optimal medical care. Time and money for the exam can instead be allocated to educational materials and supportive means. "How to" plans and doctor and community resources can be most helpful.

I find it difficult to suggest a generic schedule for health exams because both age and present health have a great influence on when the exam can be maximized for each individual. Infants should be seen monthly, older folks perhaps yearly. Healthy, active adults with minimal or no comorbidities (associated high blood pressure, diabetes, arthritis, obesity, etc.) need this encounter less frequently. The PHE has the potential to effect patient health and healthcare costs for the individual, the healthcare industry, and society as a whole. Next time you visit your doctor, ask him when you should get together and talk about the future of your health.

BOTTOM LINE: The PHE has little value unless lifestyle issues are addressed.

# THE ENDOTHELIUM

There must be something that pulls all of this together; maybe something expressed with simple words and not too much scientific jargon, but which at the same time explains what this whole story is about. Because health is such a multifaceted subject, I will only explain the end result of where the damage occurs from indiscretions and bad health choices.

Let us remind ourselves that the main focus concerning health is the cardiovascular system. Consider these statistics from the Heart Foundation:

- Heart disease is the number one cause of death for both men and women in the United States, claiming approximately 1 million lives annually.
- Every 33 seconds, someone in the United States dies from cardiovascular disease.
- More die of heart disease than of AIDS and all cancers combined.
- By 2020, heart disease will be the leading cause of death throughout the world.
- This year, more than 920,000 Americans will have a heart attack; nearly half of them will occur without prior symptoms or warning signs.[42]

The whole story about cardiovascular disease and the cause revolves around the endothelium of the vessels. Endothelium is the single-cell lining of each of the arteries, veins, and capillaries. To give you a vision of the magnitude of this system, if you laid all of the body's endothelium from every vessel flat, it would cover five tennis courts. The endothelium is the largest organ in the body, weighing five times more than the heart.

The function and chemical compounds produced in the endothelium are extensive. I will mention only one of them by name: nitric oxide (NO). Nitric oxide is involved in the relaxation and constriction of the vessels. Lesser amounts of nitric oxide than normal result in stiffening of the vessels, which leads to high blood pressure. Other chemicals produced by the endothelium have to do with clotting and plaque build-up, protection, and the general reparative process that goes into maintaining vessel integrity.

Let's talk now about disease and endothelial dysfunction. The following diseases injure the endothelium:
1. Diabetes (high blood sugar)
2. Hypertension (high blood pressure)

---

[42] http://www.theheartfoundation.org/heart-disease-facts/heart-disease-statistics/

3. Abnormal cholesterol: Elevated triglycerides, low HDL, high LDL, or "bad" cholesterol
4. Obesity
5. Smoking
6. Sedentary lifestyle
7. Other less important diseases and malfunctioning blood components

Many patients have more than one of these diseases. It's common, for instance, to have diabetes, high blood pressure, and abnormal cholesterol. One often begets another.

When the endothelium becomes maladaptive, or dysfunctional, the following things often happen: clot formation, platelet aggregation, loss of nitric oxide (the ability of the vessel to constrict and relax). The wall of the vessel itself becomes thickened and builds additional cells, often filled with fat and oxidized substances.

Organs are affected and we begin to see heart attacks, central nervous system circulatory inadequacy and clots (strokes), blindness from retinal disease and loss of kidney function—even bringing the patient into end-stage renal (kidney) disease with a high probability of dialysis. Peripheral vascular disease of the legs can occur, and the large vessel in the abdomen weakens.

BOTTOM LINE: Though death is inevitable, maintaining a healthy endothelium can lessen the onset of disease and slow down the aging process.

# COMING OUT OF THE EGG

George A. Sheehan was a 20th century physician and author best known for his writings about the sport of running. He was a track star in college, and later became a cardiologist. His book *Running & Being: The Total Experience* became a *New York Times* Best Seller.

Sheehan's article "A Neophyte at Every Age" intrigued me, and I still have a copy of it. His analysis of aging is well expressed when he quotes Chamfort, the French aphorist: "Man enters every age of his life as a neophyte. Adolescence was a mystery; so was age 20." I wonder, in the beginning, what does one know about being a husband and then a father, or wife and mother? With most of us, those "in the trenches" years foster confidence and competence. As the parental stage winds down (although it never completely winds down), the desire to embrace the "rest and relaxation" stage of one's life becomes stronger and within our grasp. Then, as Chamfort says, "one is thrust once more into the role of beginner." Every decade has a different set of challenges, needing a different set of answers. Perhaps the questions pile up faster than the answers do. Some people just seem to be able to propel themselves into the next year, the next decade, the next challenge. For some, it seems to be effortless.

Sheehan records, "No sense in dwelling on the past or wondering about the future. I have to resist the tendency that comes with age; I cannot waste my time on memories of the past—being old is different from being middle-aged as being single is from being married. Many who enter this stage dislike it." We cannot presume that success in one stage of life will be repeated in the next.

In his book *Life Cycle Completed*, Erik Erikson showed how challenging making this transition can be. He points out that very specific virtues and abilities are essential in each of these stages, as are particular strengths that are characteristically dominant or hidden during certain periods of life. We discover assets we never knew we had.

Sheehan says, "I enter this new country understanding that my life will be different and difficult. I entered my 70s as a beginner—a new man taking up a new game. Coming out of the egg and looking around is a bewildering experience."[43]

It's best to forget the past, which was probably filled with attempts (often without success) to better oneself mentally and physically, and instead look to the future and realize that, with this new commitment, that you will reach heights you have never reached before.

Many years ago, while attending a course in general medicine in San Antonio, Texas, I met an 82-year-old arthritic man. As I was finishing my noontime run, I noticed him ahead of me. His speed was limited, but I was

---

[43] *Life Cycle Completed*, Erik Erikson, W. W. Norton & Company; Extended Version edition (June 17, 1998)

amazed at this man and stopped to talk to him just before he got into his car. He had a right knee that just wouldn't straighten out, so he ran with a limp, yet his program was to exercise five times a week.

Many of us have to run with a limp, or maybe more than one limp, yet we must run—or whatever our exercise routine is—anyway. May we always have the determination to "run." What is your commitment to this new period in your life?

BOTTOM LINE: No one is immune to challenges, new experiences, or the heavy hands of aging. Every day, we have the opportunity to find the answers to new questions, or we may yet find the answers to questions that have been in our portfolio for decades.

# MAKING CHOICES

After clinical events unfold, patients and their families are too often left feeling that they would have made different choices had they "known better." That "knowing better" is best addressed by presenting information both for and against treatments, including making lifestyle changes. Knowing—and more importantly knowing *why* and *how*—to apply information makes choice that much easier, and actually more accurate.

Probably the most important challenge I am going to present you with will involve making choices. We make significant choices every day. As you make commitments and formulate goals while reading this book, you should gain enough information to define your goals and how you will reach them. You will be given choices about how you want to handle your health, rather than my insistence on one rigid program fitting everyone's needs. Choose what you can successfully use.

The way people choose is really very complicated. The correct approach is that patients and their physicians work together in making medical decisions. Making choices is profoundly based on hope and predicted outcome. If we focus on offering hope, we lay out an optimistic pattern. If we focus on difficult-to-overcome risk factors, we may present the downside of the problem and therapy, and as a result, choices may become more aggressive or even incur side effects, and may result in less than optimal outcomes.

In medicine, choices should always be based on benefit versus risk. With something simple, like an x-ray or lab test, the physician should give the patient the risk versus benefits scenario. The risk isn't really the pain from the needle stick or worrying about excess irradiation from a relatively simple x-ray of an extremity. It is what one does with the information delivered by the test or procedure. This may never have crossed your mind, but what if the test comes back abnormal, even though there is really nothing wrong? That happens not infrequently; it's called a false positive result. Another question one might ask: "Are the doctor and patient willing to act on the information, and will the resultant information change the diagnosis or treatment?"

Much more significant are choices that involve serious diagnoses, for instance, how are we going to treat a particular kind of cancer?

When it comes to lifestyle changes, choices are often made in the context of "I am doing just fine, so why change anything? I will stick with my present behavior." To patients who are healthy or feel they are healthy, disability and death seem remote relative to their current health status. Another person may understand that, although he is feeling well, research and opinions of experts say "that could change suddenly at any moment." Reference point: "I am at risk, and I had better do something about it now."

The need for making changes in one's lifestyle is based on extensive research, and the results of doing something about risk factors is very evident.

BOTTOM LINE: The risks of undertaking positive changes in your life are minimal, whereas the benefits are enormous!

# OVERVIEW OF OBESITY

Simply reading this book and deciding there is something worthwhile in it for you is a good first move. Positive feelings about self-improvement are called *the Eureka experience*, or discovery experience. *Eureka* is Greek for "I have found it." It is said that Archimedes shouted this phrase as he ran through the Agora of Athens proclaiming a mixed alloy success. In cartoons, it is represented by a light bulb turning on above a person's head. Psychologists call it the "aha phenomenon." It is the surprise of insight, the flash of inspiration that brings a long-sought solution.

Today is the day you will build upon the Eureka experience. The great thing about today is that it is the first day of the rest of your life. I wake up each morning grateful that I can have another opportunity to make today a better day. A bad day, to me, is an unfulfilled day. A bad day is quite normal—it is when you have several in a row that you might become concerned. Bad day, bad week, bad month—it is all behind you, and today you and I have another opportunity to reach our potential, or at least improve upon yesterday.

Improvement, that is so possible! Don't let yesterday's disappointments ruin today's potential. Some days, just a little progress is an accomplishment. Let's forget our disappointments. Let's forget the things that depress us and concentrate on those that exalt and build us up.

Whether you decide to begin your program of weight loss right now or at a set "start day" is an individual choice. Changing lifestyle is like climbing Mt. Everest. You occasionally look at the summit as you take each step, one at a time, one handhold after another. Don't look down, don't look back on your momentary failures. If you look down, it might destroy your momentum, and you might become frightened or frozen in your forward climb. The most successful person is the person who holds onto the old just as long as it is good, and grabs the new just as soon as it is better.

As children grow up and parents gradually relinquish their authority, and the adolescent prepares to leave the home, more and more self-reliance and individuality emerge, until the young adult has been prepared to assume the responsibility of self-direction. You have made significant positive changes in your life before; now you have to do it again. Deciding to lose weight or develop an exercise program is certainly leaving the status quo. Often, the status quo looks so good, so much in the comfort zone, so user friendly, that leaving home is too much to even think about. You may have one foot out the door, and your first impression is "Baby, it's cold outside!"

Looking down the vista of the years, we see no further than tomorrow noon. The veil over our eyes prevents us from seeing what the future will bring, as we misuse and mishandle our bodies, and glutton ourselves with the unimportant and harmful contents of the horn of plenty. Is this the life any of us want to live? Thomas Moffett said, "We dig our graves with our teeth." I believe that to be true.

Looking back in time, one of the strongest warnings about our health came from a U.S. Surgeon General, who stated that a failure to address obesity "could wipe out some of the gains we've made in areas such as heart disease, several forms of cancer, and other chronic health problems." Their efforts, plus others with like vision, have not produced the desired effect.

To put the whole process in perspective and give it a more down-home feel, let's talk about one way of visualizing obesity, and that is in the years of life lost (YLL). YLL is defined as the difference between the number of years a person would be expected to live if she was not obese and the number of years she can expect to live if she is obese. That seems simple enough.

The optimal BMI in the life-lost-years comparison is approximately 23 to 25. If your BMI is 25 to 29.5 you're overweight. If your BMI is 30 or greater you're obese. Taking the extreme risk factor BMI at over 45 (that is way, way big), white men aged 20 to 30 years with severe levels of obesity are shortening their life by 13 years, and white women by 8 years (as I mentioned in the Current Health Standings chapter). For men, this could represent a 22 percent reduction in expected remaining life span.

In John Kenneth Galbraith's *The Affluent Society*, he writes, "What is called a high standard of living consists, in considerable measure, in arrangements for avoiding muscular energy, increasing sensual pleasure and for enhancing caloric intake above any conceivable nutritional requirement."[44] These words aren't that far removed from the truth. As a matter of fact, they are right on.

In 2013, Samoa Air became the world's first airline to introduce the "fat tax," which charges overweight passengers more for their seats. The airline does not fly large commercial aircraft, but rather small planes that are more susceptible to weight variances, and the Pacific island nations have some of the world's highest rates of obesity. In urban areas of Samoa, obesity plagues up to 75 percent of the population, with diabetes three times more prevalent than in rural areas. This correlation of obesity and diabetes doesn't surprise anyone.

If you think you feel threatened and violated when you pass through security, imagine being weighed on scales at the airport, like the Samoans. The U.S. airlines probably wouldn't touch this issue with a 10-foot pole because of the negative publicity and the impracticality of weighing people at the gate. Wouldn't that be a challenge—not only asking passengers to take off their seat belts and shoes, but to individually weigh each passenger passing through security. You think the lines are long now!

The Samoa Air homepage reads "We at Samoa Air are keeping airfares fair, by charging our passengers only for what they weigh. You are the master of your air fair."[45] As you might imagine, the policy has helped to raise obesity

---

[44] *The Affluent Society*, John Kenneth Galbraith, Mariner Books; 40 Anv Sub edition (October 15, 1998)
[45] http://www.samoaair.ws

awareness and improve public health. Just picture a wife talking to her husband: "Dear, we can't go to Savai'i to visit uncle Fetu until we lose 10 pounds each." I like that conversation.

Richard Feynman was an American theoretical physicist. He received the Nobel Prize in Physics in 1965 and ranked as one of the ten greatest physicists of all time. He assisted in the development of the atomic bomb during World War II. About the bomb, Feynman was convinced that man had finally invented something that he could not control and that would ultimately destroy mankind.

I wonder how closely our fast-food addiction is to "something we cannot control" and that "will ultimately destroy mankind." Our society is plagued with a disease that seems unstoppable—the collection of excess body fat.

According to Eric Schlosser's book *Fast Food Nation*, "Americans now spend more money on fast food than on higher education, personal computers, computer software, or new cars. They spend more on fast food than on movies, books, magazines, newspapers, videos, and recorded music—combined."[46]

You and I didn't create the double burger, but we still have a responsibility for it. What is that responsibility? A greater part of it is education. We still have choice, the last time I checked!

*Researchers found that the higher the BMI, the higher the risk of death. Study participants with a BMI of 30.0 to 34.9 had a 44 percent increase in risk compared to those in the 22.5 to 24.9 range. The risk increased as BMI increased. Compared to participants in the normal weight range, those with a BMI of 35.0 to 39.9 had an 88 percent increase in risk, and those with a BMI over 40 had a 250 percent increase in risk. For every 5 unit increase in BMI, the researchers observed a 31 percent increase in risk of death.*
— The American Cancer Society[47]

Who's "fat?" If you're having a hot dog and a slice of pizza (heaven forbid) at Costco and look around, you might think the answer to this question is "all of America!" Well, not quite. More than one-third of U.S. adults (34.9 percent) are obese. More than two-thirds (68.8 percent) of adults are considered to be overweight. More than 1 in 20 (6.3 percent) have extreme obesity.[48] Normal women have 130,000 calories in their body tissues and organs. Obese women have 500,000 calories stored in fat. That is a half-million calories!

The consequences of obesity and excess weight are many and are well known to most everyone, but a fact that you may have not come across concerns

---

[46] *Fast Food Nation: The Dark Side of the All-American Meal,* Eric Schlosser, Mariner Books; Reprint edition (March 13, 2012)

[47] http://www.cancer.org/cancer/news/high-bmi-linked-to-higher-risk-of-death

[48] http://frac.org/initiatives/hunger-and-obesity/obesity-in-the-us/

Maternal Body Mass Index and adverse pregnancy outcomes. Obesity often affects more than just the person with excessive weight.

Investigators of a very large study on weight consequences and fetal outcomes conducted a systematic review and meta-analysis of 43,009 total deaths and stillbirths. They studied women with BMIs of 20, 25, and 30 and concluded "Even modest increases in maternal BMI were associated with increased risk of fetal death, stillbirth, and neonatal, perinatal, and infant death. Weight management guidelines for women who plan pregnancies should take these findings into consideration to reduce the burden of fetal death, stillbirth, and infant death."[49]

Studies have shown that babies of obese mothers can be small for their gestational age or large for their gestational age, either of which puts the baby at risk for obesity and metabolic consequences.

Most of us remember the suicidal kamikaze pilots of World War II. The Japanese nationalists portrayed the kamikaze pilots as noble soldiers willing to sacrifice their lives for the country. During World War II, nearly 4,000 kamikaze pilots were killed. About 14 percent of kamikaze attacks managed to hit a ship.

You can certainly get your quick-fix, 1,300-calorie supper at a fast food drive-through, but the increased consumption of fast food will have a greater and greater impact on the populace, and many more lives will be lost than the 4,000 kamikaze pilots killed over a span of 10 months in 1944 and 1945. Is it overkill to take the analogy to a higher level and say the end result of both is suicide?

The trend of eating out is obvious to all of us. A generation ago, three-quarters of the money to buy food in the U.S. was spent on preparing meals at home. Today, about half of the money used to buy food is spent at restaurants— most of those dollars at fast food establishments. It is more expensive to eat out, yet more and more of us do just that.

What are the health challenges of the obese person? Here are just a few:

1. High blood pressure
2. High levels of blood fats
3. High LDL levels (that's bad cholesterol)
4. Coronary heart disease
5. Osteoarthritis (wearing out of knees and hips)
6. Sleep apnea
7. Dementia and Alzheimer's disease
8. Depression
9. Certain cancers: uterine, esophageal, kidney, colon[50]

Note that 70 percent of obese youth have at least one risk factor for cardiovascular disease.[51]

---

[49] JAMA April 16, 2014 Volume 311, Number 14, pg 1536-1544,

[50] http://fasinfat.org/facts-on-obesity-and-health/

[51] http://fasinfat.org/facts-on-obesity-and-health/

The word *diet* comes from the Greek word *diaita*, meaning "way of life." In the general sense, "diet" is simply what you eat. "A diet" is what we will be discussing, and "the diet" is the one you will choose.

We need direction, and I am about to give it. Why? Take a look! The consumption of food is based on a hierarchy of choices; first, does it taste good? Second, Is it easy to prepare? Third, is it affordable? And fourth, how healthy is it? The reality is, when you are dieting and eating for the blessings of good health and longevity, taste comes first. The goods news: there are foods that are tasty, easy to prepare, affordable, and healthy.

Up front, know that there will be a bit of a bump in the road. There is a tendency for weight loss to slow after the first few weeks because of reduction in energy expenditure brought about by metabolic adaptation.

**Self-Monitoring:** Self-monitoring involves some record keeping on your part. Monitor your weight, at first daily, then weekly. Keep a daily record of your physical exercise program, and keep a food diary, too, not only noting what you are eating, but your feelings at mealtimes and any food temptations. Take a good look at the times you find yourself roaming the house trying to find food to satisfy cravings. Analyze these feelings and try to develop a response that makes dieting easier.

Another behavioral therapy approach is stimulus control: learning to avoid cues that trigger unhealthy habits such as overeating and physical inactivity. Examples of stimulus control strategies involve:
- Eating only at predetermined times (like family mealtimes)
- Bringing your lunch to work to keep to a measured caloric consumption
- Getting up and moving about right after eating instead of choosing dessert

Other types of behavioral therapies include cognitive restructuring (changing negative thought patterns), problem solving (preparing strategies to deal with challenging situations), and stress management. A seemingly small item, and one that I most always suggested to patients, was to eat nothing unless it's on a plate—even a small cracker goes on a plate. This makes you conscious of what you are doing, and makes it a little more difficult to "eat and run."

**The Brute Squad:** It is always good to get the family together to form a "brute squad." The brute squad goes into every nook and cranny of your home looking for offenders to a good sound diet. They'll get the added-sugar items out of the home and help you dispose of all those packaged chips and other types of processed, sealed goodies. Check the lists in this book that mention the various foods, which should be avoided, and get rid of them. Give them to a neighbor you're not necessarily fond of.

Eating slowly has also been studied and found to be an effective tool in weight loss. A professor in the department of kinesiology at Texas Christian University in Fort Worth, Meena Shah, conducted a study on eating slowly and calorie consumption. Shah says, "Slower eating allows people to better sense their feelings of hunger and fullness."[52] Takeaways from this creative study; eat slower, take small bites, chew thoroughly, put utensils down, and pause between bites.

Professional help in losing weight increases the likelihood of success but isn't always realistic or practical. So in the meantime, I give you an assignment: Write the following list down on a piece of paper, have it laminated, and put it next to your plate at each and every meal until you have it memorized. It describes a sensible approach to eating, in addition to setting a goal amount of caloric consumption daily.

**A Sensible Approach to Eating**

1. **Volumetric approach**—start every meal with low-calorie, high-bulk whole grains, soup, or salad (e.g., oatmeal at breakfast, salad at lunch, and soup at dinner). Studies have shown this will reduce caloric intake by 100 calories at each meal—the equivalent of half a cookie.
2. **Avoid high-calorie salad dressings**—the denser will have around 150 calories per tablespoon. You can find healthier, lower-calorie dressings that only have about 20-40 calories per tablespoon.
3. **Choose diet beverages**—We see more weight gain in regular beverage drinkers compared to diet beverage drinkers. The average American drinks 20 percent of his total daily calories, and 300 calories per day come from soda; the average American eats and drinks 150 pounds of raw sugar per year (teenagers, 250 pounds per year). Remember, adding sugar to your diet is bad whether you are trying to lose weight or not.
4. **Avoid fast foods**—A Burger King Triple Whopper contains a whopping 1,230 calories.[53] Eating fast food two times a week results in a 10-pound weight gain every year and doubles the risk for diabetes.
5. **Snacking**—Snacking is typically a habit, not a dietary necessity. Avoid dry snacks sealed in a package, like candy or chips, and instead choose snacks high in fiber and water content, like fruits and vegetables.
6. **Eat a balanced diet**—Select different foods from the many categories of foods that have proven nutritional value. Check out

---

[52] http://consumer.healthday.com/vitamins-and-nutrition-information-27/dieting-to-lose-weight-health-news-195/slow-eating-curbs-calorie-intake-683524.html

[53] http://www.acaloriecounter.com/fast-food-calories.php

The World's Healthiest Foods website at
www.whfoods.com/foodstoc.php.

7. **Consume an appropriate amount of calories**—The majority of
   women should consume1200 to 1500 calories a day; men, 1500 to
   1800 calories. To get a sense of how many calories you are
   consuming a day, you can find a calorie-counting tool online,
   download an app (I suggest http://apps.usa.gov/myfood-a-
   pedia.shtml), or buy a booklet that lists calories per food type and
   amount. (See resources at the end of this book.) As an idea of how
   counting calories works, if you can eat 500 to 750 less calories a
   day than you burn, you will lose four to six pounds in a month.

Say to yourself, "I'm not afraid to confront this problem and I think I can
solve it." This attitude doesn't need to come from abundant resources; rather,
from the self-esteem of knowing you can achieve something good and important
even if it's hard to do. Personally, I have a "funny quirk": every day I think I will be
able to achieve my goals, yet at the end of day, I am not where I wanted to be.
Still, my day has not been wasted. The next day, I start all over believing in
myself that I CAN do it. As self-help author Anthony Robbins reminds us,
"Confidence breeds competence!"

BOTTOM LINE: For weight loss, women should consume 1200 to 1500 calories
a day. For men, 1500 to 1800 calories. You can get great help tracking food
selections and counting calories online, and if you're not a computer user, there
are plenty of books that will suffice.

# OBESITY AND HABITS

Do you remember hearing commands like "Clean your plate" or "If you eat your beans, you can have dessert" from your parents? As a child, were you often rewarded with food? That was commonplace at our house. If you grew up being rewarded with food, I would bet that you are probably still rewarding yourself with food. Over a period of time, that behavior becomes fairly ingrained in the hardwiring of your brain.

Every time you repeat a thought or an action, you strengthen the connection between a set of brain cells. The synapses become more aligned with one another, and connections in tandem are strengthened. Dr. Rick Hanson, a neuroscience expert and psychologist, says, "The mind and the brain are a unified system. As the brain changes, the mind changes. As the mind changes, the brain changes. This means that you can use your conscious mind to make lasting changes to your brain to bring about greater well-being and happiness in your life."[54] Neuroscientist Carla Shatz said, "Neurons that fire together, wire together."[55]

When one neuron fires, a giant sequence of activity occurs in the neurons that are tightly bound together. People's behavior today is a result of yesterday's responses. One might think of these habit-like replays as little tapes in your brain. That is why it is difficult to overcome yesterday's non-productive and often injurious habits, and why we find ourselves repeating the painful activities of yesterday.

The good news is there is enough neuroplasticity to disconnect or "rewire" these habit templates in our brains. Author Sharon Begley states, "We are not stuck with the brain we were born with but have the capacity to willfully direct which functions will flower and which will wither, which moral capacities emerge and which do not, which emotions flourish and which are stilled."[56] If we develop good habits, they will replace the bad and painful habits. This is why it is important to write down goals, roadblocks, and other things that need attention. Write them out in form of the present; make them personal and with strong meaningful affirmation.

**The point:** You can overcome some pretty bad habits if you begin with belief—belief in yourself and belief in the words of this book. One of your allies is self-talk (see the chapter about this).

The following are habits that you will want to become your mode of

---

[54] http://www.rickhanson.net/seven-facts-brain-incline-mind-joy/

[55] *The Brain That Changes Itself: Stories of Personal Triumph from the Frontiers of Brain Science*, by Norman Doidge, M.D., Penguin Books, 2007

[56] *Train Your Mind, Change Your Brain: How a New Science Reveals Our Extraordinary Potential to Transform Ourselves*, by Sharon Begley, Mac Audio, 2008

operation. Put them on your checklist of "things to do."

**New Habits**

1.  Prepare and eat your meals in the kitchen. Don't snack in the study, in front of the TV, or in bed.
2.  Don't focus on cleaning your plate; instead, clean your table and counter. Put leftovers away immediately. Food out of sight is less likely to find its way into your mouth.
3.  Always sit down and eat anything from a plate, even if it is as small as a cracker. This will help with unconscious "piecing." If you're eating with family, it also ensures that you eat your first bite together.
4.  Use a smaller dinner plate than you used to.
5.  Get up from the table as soon as you finish eating and quickly begin working on your "non-food to-do list." The destructive pattern of roaming around the kitchen looking for another morsel after you have eaten will disappear. This will take your focus off of food.

A word of warning to the newly married couple: The average weight gain in the first year of married life is 10 pounds, and it's all downhill from there. The Obesity Society also tells us that many married and single people in their late teens and early twenties gain an average of 15 to 30 pounds over five years.[57]

BOTTOM LINE: People's behavior today is a result of yesterday's responses. We have the capacity to change our hardwired bad habits with positive thinking. Immediately put into practice the new habits on this list.

---

[57] http://usatoday30.usatoday.com/news/health/2007-10-22-marriage-weight_N.htm?csp=34

# EATING OUT

If you are on a diet, eating out is always a challenge. Restaurant portions have doubled or tripled in the last two decades.[58] These days, eating more is the norm.

Even for skinny people, eating out is problematic. I am always enticed by the oversized, high-calorie, salty, fatty, fried foods that were made just for me. Oh, so tempting! Where did my resolve to be prudent when ordering food go? Almost all of us eat out frequently. According to *Christian Science Monitor*, the average American spends $232 per month eating out. This breaks down to an average of each person eating out four or five times a week.[59] This surprises me, since eating out is expensive. When folks tighten their belts, one of their options to make the paycheck stretch is to stay at home and eat something they can afford. But, such is our culture. "Sixty percent of our population has to "tighten the belt" around a waist which is just too big because they are either overweight or obese. For females, if your waist is over 34 inches, that is too big. For males, that figure is over 39 inches.

If you want to lose weight, or just create a more healthy diet, I would suggest that one of your first goals would be to stop eating out altogether for _____ weeks. You fill in the blank! If you are currently eating out infrequently, you can still pledge not to eat out at all for three or four weeks. Stopping for a while will give that extra jumpstart to your lifestyle program. After you begin to achieve success, you may reconnect with the eating-out experience, but keep it down to perhaps 50 percent of your previous schedule. When you do eat out, may I make a few suggestions?

- See if the menu posts calories. Many restaurants do. If not, make a list of the food you ate so you can check online later. Better still, before you set foot in an establishment, go online and tally the calorie count of your anticipated meal. If you have your smartphone at the restaurant, you can also go to MyFood-A-Pedia (http://apps.usa.gov/myfood-a-pedia.shtml) to check out the number of calories in your food.
- Most restaurants offer low-calorie or "lite" meals. Generally, this means they simply downsize the proportions.
- Drink lots of water with each meal.
- Eat slowly, and don't take the next bite until you have swallowed the previous morsel.
- Order a salad. Ask for dressings "on the side" so you can use only as

---

[58] http://www.nhlbi.nih.gov/health/educational/wecan/news-events/matte1.htm

[59] http://www.csmonitor.com/Business/The-Simple-Dollar/2012/0710/Common-dollars-and-sense-Eating-less-fast-food-does-a-body-good

much as you want. Dressings are notorious for having a lot of calories, so use them sparingly. A simple oil and vinegar mix tends to have fewer calories—or simply use plain vinegar.

- Appetizers are not only expensive but also deadly, in that they usually contain a lot of calories and salt.
- Avoid the bread. Refuse seconds, and don't take the firsts, either. Bread is always a killer for me. A hard roll contains about 168 calories, a brown-crusted roll about 128.
- Drinks can contain a lot of calories, and if refills are no extra cost, that can be a big calorie hog. I would suggest avoiding milk altogether. If your routine is to drink tea, get it unsweetened or use artificial sweetener.
- Choose the same kinds of dishes you have at home (or should be having): vegetables, fruits, low-fat dairy products, and whole grains. If you are having meat, make sure it is lean. There is much to be said about eating a dish without meat. Make some of your eating out experiences plant-based, or more to the point, vegetarian. Note that fish is generally the exception to this, and often a healthy option.
- As a rule, don't eat desserts. They are packed with calories, and all they do is take you beyond satiety and make you feel stuffed and disappointed in your dietary resolve.
- Select steamed, broiled, or grilled dishes instead of those that are fried or sautéed. Foods that are breaded are higher in calories.
- Order fruit and steamed vegetables without butter or sauce.
- Choose steamed or broiled fish and ask for lemon and fresh herbs for seasonings.
- When you are through, you're through. Have the waiter take your plate. Leaving uneaten food in front of you is fatal. It's too tempting to pick at it. Again, another one of my own weaknesses.

Once you achieve a certain level of determination, it won't be that hard to eat out. There will be challenges and disappointments. The ancient Norse crest has a pickaxe as an emblem, and the motto reads, "Either I will find a way or make one."

BOTTOM LINE: Eating out is dangerous to your health. When eating out, I strongly recommend you make a copy of the above suggestions and follow them closely.

# SELF-TALK, A TOOL FOR SELF-IMPROVEMENT

We have 100 billion neurons in our brains, with 50,000 connections to each one of those neurons. This is an enormous network for storage of information and reaction to life around us. When we have negative thoughts or experiences, they become hardwired into our brains and eventually become our masters, in spite of our knowing the negative consequences of our actions and reactions. Sometimes, our negative behaviors stick as if they were made of Velcro. We must override these pathways and informational packets.

This seemingly overwhelming challenge can be facilitated by what is called self-talk. The self-talk strategy can be used to improve interaction with your environment. This form of therapy places you in an active role as you make changes in your life.

Self-talk therapy and techniques are nearly as old as time. Buddha perhaps best summarized self-talk therapy: "We are what we think. All that we are arises with our thoughts. With our thoughts, we make our world."

Then there's Proverb 23:7: "For he that thinketh in his heart, so is he."

How we feel, and therefore how we react to things, is based on our thoughts. Self-talk draws on this simple idea to show us how the way we talk to ourselves—our internal dialogue—plays a large role in how we feel and how we perceive our experiences.

The following are the key sequences of experience and emotion-stimulus, self-talk, and emotion. First, there is a stimulus: something happens in our environment that affects us. Then, we try to determine just what this stimulus means. We do this through self-talk (internal dialogue through the "clearinghouse" of our brains/emotion) or through a set of predetermined rules we have set up. Rules are simply shortcuts to self-talk, so that in reoccurring situations we can respond more quickly, with a predetermined answer, to what a stimulus means. We can liken this to a reflex; it is automatic. This "clearinghouse" in our brain will decide how we feel about any specific experience.

Let me give you a couple of concrete examples. Two people are waiting at the same traffic light in separate cars. The first person sees the red light and thinks to himself. "This really is bad! Here's another couple of minutes taken from my life! What did I do to deserve this?" This person gets very upset and frustrated. He has interpreted the red light personally and is pained by this experience.

The second person notices the red light and thinks to himself, "This is great! Now I have time to take a big breath, an opportunity to check my tie in the mirror." This person has interpreted the same red-light stop as an opportunity. Under the same exact circumstances, he has a totally different experience based on the interpretation of the event created through his self-talk.

Another example: You are trying to lose weight, but the constant desire to grab a bite of this or that is very real. A positive approach to self-talk could be, "I'll still be hungry after consuming this morsel, and it will serve no positive function for me to eat it; I am stronger than the desire to eat." At every opportunity throughout the day, tell yourself the truth: "I am a worthwhile person and am in control of my life." Will you always succeed? No! But that is part of self-talk—to be unrelenting in positive thoughts and to constantly reassure yourself that winning is about getting up one more time than you are knocked down.

Your brain will come up with an answer for any question that you ask with sincerity. The brain does not determine if the answer is true or false; it simply provides possible answers based on the questions. If you ask yourself, "Why am I so stupid?" your mind will quickly obey and generate a multitude of reasons as to why you are so stupid. On the other hand, if you ask yourself "In which ways am I smart?" your mind will begin to generate several possible reasons.

Self-talk therapy has enormous potential. The better we understand ourselves and others, the more balanced, understanding, and influential we are.

Interested in learning more about self-talk? Read *Awaken the Giant Within* by Anthony Robbins.

BOTTOM LINE: Self-talk rewires neural pathways. Positive self-talk needs attention, needs to be frequent if not constant, and changes bad habits into good habits.

# CANCER CAUSED BY POOR LIFESTYLE

Sedentary lifestyle is the culprit; regular physical activity is the solution. Regular physical activity reduces the risk of many types of cancers by augmenting weight control, and reduces the chances of colorectal and breast cancer by other processes as well. Those in the know tell us that exercise should be of moderate intensity, and many authorities suggest a program of 150 minutes per week in aerobic exercise, which is less than an hour daily. I would suggest, optimally, one hour each day.

Dr. Walter Willett, chair of the department of nutrition at the Harvard School of Public Health, tells us that "Increasingly intensive strategies will be needed to reverse the obesity epidemic, and actions are needed in many sectors and at all levels of society."[60] That is a daunting task, but needs to be addressed. You have joined the ranks of the faithful and will add strength to help it all happen!

Being simply overweight is less worrisome than being obese. As a reminder, body mass index (BMI) is calculated as weight in kilograms divided by height in meters squared, and overweight is a BMI of 25 to 30. A BMI of 30 to 40 is obesity. The evidence for obesity increasing the risk for cancers is overwhelming. A dose-response is present, meaning, the more excessive the body fat, the worse the health prospects.

Excess body fat increases the risk for cancers of the esophagus, pancreas, colon, kidney, breast, and uterus. High consumption of red meat, especially processed meat, is associated with a risk for colorectal cancer.

We are constantly waving the flag of the tobacco and cancer connection, but weight is also a big player—pun intended.

"Although the risks of cancer for an individual who is overweight or obese are not as great as they are for a tobacco smoker, in the United States and some other countries, the much higher prevalence of overweight and obesity than smoking means that the numbers of cancer deaths caused by these two factors are now similar," Dr. Willett comments.[61]

He points out that added sugar in beverages, like soda, is a particularly important contributing factor to the unhealthy lifestyle so many Americans have assumed. One of the ways we can attempt to stem the tide: "The scientific evidence base to support soda taxation has become much more solid in the past several years, and this should be pursued vigorously as a public health strategy," he comments. He further address the beverage issue by stating, "In the United States, political gridlock and the powerful influences of the food and beverage

---

[60] http://www.iarc.fr/en/publications/books/wcr/Willett.pdf

[61] http://www.iarc.fr/en/publications/books/wcr/Willett.pdf

industries often make national actions impossible,"[62] Local solutions often seem more effective, such as PTAs banning soda machines in schools. As an example of this type of strategy, in April 7, 2011, Mayor Thomas M. Menino issued an executive order requiring Boston City departments to take steps to phase out the sale, advertising, and promotion of sugary beverages on city-owned property.

BOTTOM LINE: In addition to incorporating physical activity into our lifestyle, treatment of overweight and obesity must be a high priority for cancer prevention.

---

[62] http://www.iarc.fr/en/publications/books/wcr/Willett.pdf

# NATIONAL WEIGHT CONTROL REGISTRY

The National Weight Control Registry (NWCR), established in 1994 by Rena Wing, Ph.D. from Brown Medical School, and James O. Hill, Ph.D. from the University of Colorado, is the largest prospective investigation of long-term successful weight loss maintenance. We can learn much from what their research has to tell us. You need to put your heart into this one. It is chock full of helpful information and even reinforcement directed toward *you*. You are there somewhere, just look.

The NWCR was developed to identify behavioral and psychological characteristics and strengths of individuals who have succeeded at long-term weight loss. Detailed questionnaires and annual follow-up surveys are used to obtain the necessary information for the study.

Participants in the National Weight Control Registry found that those who had maintained a significant weight loss reported improvements in not only their physical health, but also their energy levels, general mood, and self-confidence.

## Statistical Analysis of the NWCR Program

1. 80 percent of those studied are women, 20 percent men.
2. The average woman is 45 years of age and currently weighs 145 pounds.
3. The average man is 49 years of age and currently weighs 190 pounds.
4. Registry members have lost an average of 66 pounds and have kept it off for 5.5 years.
5. Weight loss range: from 30 to 300 pounds
6. Some have lost weight rapidly; others have lost weight very slowly—for up to 14 years.
7. 45 percent of registry participants lost the weight on their own, while 55 percent lost it with the help of some type of program (i.e. Weight Watchers).
8. 98 percent modified their food intake in some way to lose the weight.
9. 94 percent increased their physical activity, most frequently with walking.[63]

Other characteristics common to most of these people include keeping accurate food records, exercising 60-90 minutes each day, weighing themselves regularly, and seeing their healthcare provider on a regular basis.

Keeping your weight down, after the valiant effort in losing it, is a task comparable to painting the Golden Gate Bridge, in that it never ceases. It is a

---

[63] http://www.nwcr.ws

daily endeavor. "Once an alcoholic, always an alcoholic", and "once a foodaholic, always a foodaholic." This isn't AA, but here are some of the ways in which study participants keep the weight off:

1. Continuing to maintain a low calorie, low fat diet
2. Continuing high levels of activity
3. 90 percent exercise, on average, about one hour per day
4. 78 percent eat breakfast every day.
5. 75 percent weigh themselves at least once a week.
6. 62 percent watch less than 10 hours of TV per week.

There you have it, the wide variety of ways in which success occurs, and sticks. Look at each item, noting where you presently stand and what options you have in selecting your own weight loss program.

Keeping it off is the ultimate success. The death of most successful maintenance programs is the failure to maintain previous behavioral changes that helped achieve success in the first place.

From the viewpoint of success, weight-loss maintainers lost an average of 37 pounds and maintained it for over seven years. They had ongoing self-styled behavioral strategies to control dietary fat intake. Remember, in keeping it off, cutting down on fat trumps a low carbohydrate diet.

Physical activity is a very important factor in keeping weight off. Recent recommendations advise 60 to 90 minutes to prevent weight regain. In the study, physical activity was more frequent and more strenuous, with longer periods of exercise. Participants also weighed themselves more regularly. Consistent self-monitoring of weight is a key component of successful weight loss maintenance. Studies show that more frequent weighing is associated with lower BMI. After entering the program, weight gain at one-year follow-ups was significantly greater for participants whose self-weighing frequency decreased between baseline and one year, compared with those whose frequency increased or remained the same.

I would suggest weighing yourself one morning a week. Participants in the study who decreased their frequency of self-weighing were more likely to report increases in their percentage of caloric intake from fat.

**The Basic 10 About Weight Loss**

1. You're never too old or too obese to begin a weight loss program.
2. Slower weight loss is more likely to be successful. Think small at first. If you have 80 pounds to lose, try to first lose five to ten pounds over one to two months, then bite off another small chunk.
3. Establish good eating habits, and stick to them for the rest of your life.
4. You are more likely to be successful if you involve others—family, or even a program.
5. Decreased total caloric consumption over caloric expenditures will

cause weight loss. For maintaining weight, focus on decreasing your fat intake unless your physician directs otherwise.

6. Eat three smaller meals a day. If you have to snack, it should always be with lower calorie fruits (i.e. apples) or unlimited vegetables (i.e. carrots, celery).

7. Eliminate or drastically cut down on sedentary activities, particularly TV watching.

8. Increase your physical activity to 30 minutes or more daily. If immobility problems prevent you from doing aerobic exercise, do what you can.

9. Weigh yourself once a week. Don't play the daily "scale game," allowing yourself that extra serving of potatoes and dessert every time you lose a pound or if you're not losing and not meeting your goals, skip a meal.

10. Never give up! The winner is the one who gets up one more time than he falls down.

# BEHAVIOR TIPS

This chapter is a practical way for you to keep track of your own progress in your attempts to change your behavior around eating as the months go by. I would suggest that you either copy this page or just write in the book. After the first month, make a mark in red in the parenthesis of each of the 8 activities. After the next month, use black or blue just below, then maybe yellow after the third month. This will be helpful in comparing your progress.

These are eight assignments for approaching your weight loss effort—certainly not all of the ammunition available, but a good start. These eight items should be a minimum in your program. If you execute them regularly and effectively, success will be yours. Not only will you lose weight, but I will give you a five-star rating for effort!

1. When hit by cravings to eat, do something else.
   Excellent ( )   Good ( )      Fair ( ) Poor ( )      Impossible ( )
2. Be the slowest eater. Don't fill the fork before you're finished chewing.
   Excellent ( )   Good ( )      Fair ( ) Poor ( )      Impossible ( )
3. Enjoy salads without dressing; try lemon instead.
   Excellent ( )   Good ( )      Fair ( ) Poor ( )      Impossible ( )
4. Learn contents, so you can easily calculate caloric value and fat content.
   Excellent ( )   Good ( )      Fair ( ) Poor ( )      Impossible ( )
5. Learn alternative cooking styles. A fried egg has twice the calories that a boiled egg has.
   Excellent ( )   Good ( )      Fair ( ) Poor ( )      Impossible ( )
6. Budget your calories before and after special occasions.
   Excellent ( )   Good ( )      Fair ( ) Poor ( )      Impossible ( )
7. Store "high-risk" foods away from easy access. Eliminate most, if not all.
   Excellent ( )   Good ( )      Fair ( ) Poor ( )      Impossible ( )
8. Develop a substitution list; identify high-calorie foods and find substitutes with half the calories.
   Excellent ( )   Good ( )      Fair ( ) Poor ( )      Impossible ( )

## Shopping Tips

Shopping tips are simple but effective guidelines. There are many, but you won't necessarily face every single one of these challenges when trying to lose weight. However, if you can get clear in your mind what is in the way of your success, you will become more motivated to change behavior.

1. Purchase fresh foods rather than processed foods.
2. Shop after eating, not while you are hungry.
3. Stick to a prepared shopping list.
4. Choose plain canned or frozen vegetables rather than those with sauces.
5. Carefully scrutinize claims that a product is "low-calorie," "lite," or "healthy."
6. Choose cuts of meat that have the least amount of visible fat, and trim this visible fat off of meats. "Prime" beef has more saturated fat; step down and buy a lesser grade.

BOTTOM LINE: Discipline yourself to read guidelines frequently and follow them closely. They are excellent allies in losing weight.

# BMI

If you do much reading about health, you will frequently run across the abbreviation BMI, or body mass index. BMI is a measurement of body fat based on height and weight. BMI is actually a calculation made by taking the person's weight in kilograms divided by his height (meters squared). Seems complicated, and it is, but there are simple BMI calculators available online.

Using the National Heart, Lung, and Blood Institute's terminology:
Underweight = <18.5
Normal weight = 18.5–24.9
Overweight = 25–29.9
Obesity = BMI of 30 or greater[64]

Grade 1 obesity is defined as a BMI of 30 to less than 35; grade 2 obesity, a BMI of 35 to less than 40; and grade 3 obesity, a BMI of 40 or greater.

How much weight do you need to lose to be where you should be? If your BMI is 25 or higher, you could decrease your health risks by losing some weight. Losing even 5 to 10 percent could have a significant impact. The amount you need to lose to get your BMI below 25 depends on your height, for example:

- If you are 5'5" and your BMI is 27, you need to lose 13 pounds to get your BMI below 25. If your BMI is 30, you need to lose 31 pounds to get your BMI below 25.
- If you are 6' and your BMI is 27, you need to lose 16 pounds to get your BMI below 25. If your BMI is 30, you need to lose 38 pounds to get your BMI below 25.

BMI is a good way to determine the risk of premature death and aids in the measurement of progress in changing one's behavior.

"The optimal BMI, associated with the least number of years of life lost or greatest longevity, is approximately 23 to 25 for whites and 23 to 30 for blacks. For any given degree of overweight, younger adults generally have greater number of years of life lost, than did older adults." — *Journal of the American Medical Association (JAMA)*, January 8, 2003[65]

---

[64] http://www.nhlbi.nih.gov/guidelines/obesity/BMI/bmicalc.htm
[65] *Journal of the American Medical Association (JAMA)*, January 8, 2003[65]: pg187-193

# WAIST CIRCUMFERENCE

Measuring waist circumference is another tool we have to determine risk for cardiovascular disease. If a person is normal in all other aspects, including body mass index, an increased central measurement (waist circumference) adds one additional risk factor to the patient's propensity for heart disease, stroke, renal disease, etc.

Technically, the waist circumference is measured at a level midway between the lowest rib and the hipbone, at the end of expiration (breathing out). Actually, I measure waist circumference at the level of the belly button. If a person has an "overhanging" belly, measure the waist circumference part way up the protuberant fat, where the belly button should be.

Women should have a waist measurement of less than 35 inches, while men should have a measurement of less than 40 inches. The size of a person's waist or waist circumference, if abnormal, indicates abdominal obesity, also called central obesity. Abdominal fat produces things we don't want to have, such as free fatty acids, which are turned into triglycerides. The triglycerides add to the burden of vascular disease. Excess abdominal fat is a risk factor for developing heart disease and other obesity-related diseases. The National, Heart, Lung and Blood Institute (NHLBI)'s standards indicate that men with a waist circumference greater than 102 cm (40 in) and women with a waist circumference greater than 88 cm (35 in) are at higher risk.[66]

Of course, abdominal fat, which causes the increase in abdominal girth, is more common in men. There is also a genetic tendency for the depositing of fat in the abdomen in some ethnic groups, such as Asians. For Asian folks, the upper limit of body mass index (BMI) is 23, and 25 in Caucasians. The most accurate way to measure abdominal fat is by computed tomography (CT), but it is very expensive, and the quick and inexpensive use of the tape measure is really all we need.

Glycogen is the most immediate releasable source of energy, so the body's propensity when confronted with extra calories is to convert those nutrients to glycogen. Glycogen is made and stored in the liver, but excess is "kicked out" and is stored in subcutaneous tissue as fat. That fat is then deposited around the abdominal organs. The most difficult fat to release for usage is abdominal fat, thus explaining why the gut circumference is slow to decline when weight loss is undertaken. So, as you lose weight, be patient with your belly.

To get a more accurate perception of abdominal fat, think of the fat around your abdominal organs as an organ in itself. Fat is not inert, but alive and kicking. This "organ" produces elements such as IL-6 (which promotes inflammation),

---

[66] http://www.nhlbi.nih.gov/health/public/heart/obesity/lose_wt/risk.htm

PAI-1 (which promotes atherosclerosis, or hardening of the arteries),and hsCRP, which also promotes inflammation.

It stands to reason that those with a bigger waist circumference—and more abdominal fat—generate more inpatient charges.

Obviously, weight reduction is the answer to the problem of abnormal waist circumference. It is tough to do, but nonetheless, necessary. Reduction in waist circumference by two to three inches can reduce risk for type 2 diabetes by 60 percent, and that is nothing to scoff at!

BOTTOM LINE: Abdominal fat is an active, "in the game" organ constantly exerting its negative metabolic effects. When you bump into the wall and your belly hits it before your nose, you have a big time problem.

# NON-EXERCISE ACTIVITY THERMOGENESIS

The three components of daily energy expenditure are:
1. **Basal metabolic rate** — The energy you expend by simply existing, without exercise or activity, which accounts for about 60 to 70 percent of daily caloric expenditure
2. **Thermic effect of food** — The heat given off or calories burned during the breakdown of ingested food, which accounts for about 10 percent of daily caloric expenditure
3. **Activity thermogenesis** — The calories used during the activities of daily living, including exercise and non-exercise activity

Within activity thermogenesis, we have non-exercise-related energy expenditure (NEAT): the burning of calories beyond just existing in the awakened state, but not including the calories you burn with an exercise program. NEAT is pivotal in the regulation of human energy expenditure and body weight regulation.

Studies suggest that NEAT may differ by as much as 2,000 calories per day between two adults of similar size and weight, because of differing occupations and leisure-time activities. We also know that lean individuals naturally tend to be more active than obese or overweight individuals. Obese individuals, overall, stand and ambulate two and a half hours per day less than lean individuals.[67] However, surprisingly, when obese or overweight individuals lose weight, their activity levels generally do not increase. This suggests that there is a genetic component to non-exercise physical activity. This is not offered as an excuse, just a fact that may help us understand our difficulty in trying to lose weight.

What does all this mean and how can we use it to our advantage? First, doctors should provide patients with a choice of physical activities. Again, you are best able to choose what might work for you. The exercise types you choose will most likely insure a higher compliance rate. I like to recommend activities that have immediate rewards, such as walking while listening to music, as well as convenience. It's important to identify barriers to maintaining an exercise routine.

Make a list of which habits prevent effective NEAT calorie burning, such as watching TV in your spare time or always taking the shortest distance from point A to point B. Then, list all the things that you can do to increase your NEAT, things like:
- Choosing to stand up rather than sitting
- Walking around a little more
- Taking the stairs once in a while

---

[67] http://atvb.ahajournals.org/content/26/4/729.full

- Even doing things like hand-washing your dishes or getting out to do yard work more often
- Choose walking rather than driving

I think you get the idea. These are fairly pointed, impactful suggestions, but you may have other ideas. I strongly urge you to get pencil and paper and do as instructed.

BOTTOM LINE: Anything but sitting or sleeping is NEAT—I mean, really neat. You're "neater" when you purposefully go out of your way to move that body of yours. Think "move" in everything you do.

# PLANT-BASED DIETS AFFECT WEIGHT LOSS

A recent study out of the University of South Carolina suggests that vegetarian and vegan diets, which don't emphasize counting calories, lead to more weight loss at eight weeks and six months than diets, which include meat. Doctors have long suspected that plant-based diets facilitated weight reduction, but it's nice to have that hunch backed up with good research.

The New DIETs (Dietary Interventions to Enhance the Treatments for Weight Loss) study is the first study to directly compare meat, vegan, and vegetarian diets without a specific calorie-ingestion protocol. They randomly assigned 63 adults (mean age of 49 years and mean BMI of 35) to one of five diets: vegan, vegetarian, pesco-vegetarian, semi-vegetarian, and omni-vegetarian. Each diet emphasized low-glycemic-index and low-fat foods, but did not require caloric restriction.

**Vegan Diet**—No meat, poultry, fish, dairy, or eggs. The diet includes an associated ethical philosophy about animals and their use.

**Vegetarian Diet**—Abstaining from the consumption of meat, including poultry and seafood.

**Pesco-vegetarian Diet**—A diet that includes fish or other seafood, but not the flesh of other animals.

**Semi-vegetarian Diet**—Vegetarian diet with limited red meat and poultry— less than once a month for red meat and once a week for poultry.

**Omni-vegetarian diet**—Short for "omnivore," an omni-vegetarian is a person who is non-vegetarian.

The results showed that, at eight weeks, the groups eating a plant-based diet without any meat had lost an average of eight to ten pounds. Those consuming some meat had lost an average of five pounds.

At six months, the following was observed:

- Vegans had lost about 7 percent of their body weight.
- The semi-vegetarian group had lost about 4 percent of their body weight.
- The pesco-vegetarian group had lost about 3 percent of their body weight.
- The omnivorous group had also lost about 3 percent of their body

weight.[68]

We know that vegetarians have the lowest BMIs, the lowest prevalence of type 2 diabetes, and the lowest amount of weight gain over time. In an overview about this study, ClinicalTrials.gov states: "In addition, vegetarians have significantly better metabolic risk factors as compared to non-vegetarians."[69]

Complete adherence to an unrefined plant-based diet will be one of your best tools for losing weight. As Dr. Campbell points out below, you can in fact "eat all you want" and still lose weight. The value of a plant-based diet is extensively discussed in his book, *The China Study*.

BOTTOM LINE: A vegetarian diet (plant-based) is a proven tool in a successful weight-loss program. If you need to lose weight, you can't do better than this diet.

---

[68] http://www.consultant360.com/exclusives/vegetarian-diets-affect-weight-loss
[69] http://clinicaltrials.gov/show/NCT01742572

# OBESITY: LONG-TERM STRATEGY TO PREVENT WEIGHT GAIN

At the end of the day, the successful strategy of "eat less and exercise more" is still sound advice for preventing long-term weight gain.

Researchers in a study called "Changes in Diet and Lifestyle and Long-Term Weight Gain in Women and Men" involved 120,877 men and women who, initially, were free of chronic disease and not obese. At four-year intervals from1986 to 2006, 1991 to 2003, and 1986 to 2006, lifestyle factors and weight change were evaluated. The results were very telling: those being studied gained an average of 3.35 pounds within each four-year period. This information can be a valuable aid in mapping out an effective program for keeping "ugly pounds" off.

The New England Journal of Medicine article about this study states, "On the basis of increased daily servings of individual dietary components, four-year weight change was most strongly associated with the intake of potato chips (1.69 lb), potatoes (1.28 lb), sugar-sweetened beverages (1.00 lb), unprocessed red meats (0.95 lb), and processed meats (0.93 lb) and was inversely associated with the intake of vegetables (–0.22 lb), whole grains (–0.37 lb), fruits (–0.49 lb), nuts (–0.57 lb), and yogurt (–0.82 lb)."[70]

Now, I want you to take your pen or pencil out and make a list with a "bad guys" column and a "good guys" column, and write the above information on this list. Put this list on your refrigerator.

Of course, other lifestyle factors besides diet were examined in the study, and as one might suppose, physical activity results in weight loss, sleeping too much or not enough (less than six or more than eight hours of sleep) put pounds on participants, and television watching has an adverse effect.

In facing the future, don't get weighed down with discouragement. When you get discouraged, think of Noah. He was told by the Lord to preach His gospel. He did it for three years, then the Lord drowned all his contacts! But he persevered and never complained about cleaning all the animal pens and birdcages.

When it comes to satisfying the overzealous appetite, remember that "no" is a complete sentence.

BOTTOM LINE: Multiple lifestyle factors are needed to effectively lose weight. Specific dietary and lifestyle factors are independently associated with long-term weight gain. It is altogether appropriate to develop strategies to keep the weight off early on.

---

[70] http://www.nejm.org/doi/full/10.1056/NEJMoa1014296

# THE ART OF MEDICINE

The art of medicine, has it disappeared? Is it important to know the answer to this question when you go to your caregiver for advice about your health? First of all, what really is medicine—traditionally and as we know it today?

Medicine is a science built upon evidence-based information; certainly, the administration of care becomes *the art of medicine*. The object of medical science is to study disease. Centuries ago, there were no significant "studies," or even those interested in gathering data from clinical experience, so the science of medicine was lacking. It wasn't that there weren't skilled practitioners (relatively speaking), but listening and holding the hands of the ill and dying were about all that they could do. These attributes—being able to console, exhibit compassion, and show understanding—are still necessary to be a "complete" physician. And in modern times, the science of medicine takes advantage of ever-growing, marvelous technology to allow us to look into every nook and cranny of the body, from the brain to the blood.

*Cecil Textbook of Medicine* states:

> *Medicine is a profession that incorporates science and scientific methods with the art of being a physician. The art of tending to the sick is as old as humanity itself. Compared with its long and generally distinguished history of caring and comforting, the scientific basis of medicine is remarkably recent. But the science of medicine changes with the progress of science and changing concepts from time to time. So, the art of medicine, or compassion, care, sympathy etc., are the building blocks of the practice of the science of medicine.[71]*

The art of medicine is essentially composed of the clinical skills of listening and advocacy brought to bear in the doctor/patient encounter. In early times, medicine was primarily an art. As science has propelled us into a different world of medicine, that art has been minimized. Along with the rapid advances in technology, there has been a corresponding decline in the human traits of healthcare providers, changing the once sacred doctor-patient relationship.

In *Science and the Art of Medicine, Journal of Indian Academy of Clinical Medicine*, Hedge has expressed similar concern over the issue. He states:

---

[71] *Cecil Textbook of Medicine -- 2-Volume Set, Text with Continually Updated Online Reference*, Lee Goldman and Dennis Ausiello, Saunders, 22nd edition, January 2004

*The art of clinical medicine is dying in the present teaching set up with high-tech gadgets. In the field of medical education these days, there is not much emphasis on the art of medicine. In only one university in the world, at Brisbane, students are recruited into medical schools after they have learned music, philosophy etc., a very good beginning indeed.[72]*

Philip Overby, M.D., M.A. states: "Today, doctors are both more powerful and more deaf. They are far less helpless in the face of suffering, yet they often cannot hear the cries that evoke no possibility of remedy."[73] That statement should get your attention!

With computers, stacks of paperwork, increasing high-tech procedures which distance patients from the doctors, legal entanglements, and the high price of medical care, it is easy to lose touch with the patient. When I say "lose touch" I mean that quite literally.

Curing the patient is the ultimate goal of the doctor, but often we as physicians can't cure every patient, and we particularly can't cure that patient now, or tomorrow, or next week. It may take a lifetime. But we can care about the patient now, tomorrow, next week, and beyond. Caring is best done with a sound doctor-patient relationship in place, where the doctor exhibits empathy and the time-honored physical exam is undertaken. Evidence-based medicine is beginning to report that such things as physician breast exams and checks for prostate masses as a screening tool are no longer necessary, because they don't lead to increased longevity. Putting our "hands on" is a diagnostic tool I hate to see scrapped, but that is what is happening.

The art of medicine involves not only touching the patient physically, but touching the patient emotionally. Getting into the patient's heart is the true measure of how effectively a physician has performed in the medical arena. More and more, whether right or wrong, the average physician does not lay hands upon the patient, but rather sits in front of the computer and scans, searches, and enters in data. We draw data from around the world but ignore the patient in front of us. That isn't the way we should be practicing medicine. Devices distract us from who we really are as caregivers. After all, why listen to the heart when echocardiograms can be done? Why look at the whites of a patient's eyes when we can check their bilirubin by a simple blood test? Why listen to the chest when we can do a chest CT scan? I believe that the art of medicine, quickly fading away, means being honest with patients and letting them know even when we don't have answers.

We have all heard someone say, "That doctor has a good bedside manner," or conversely, "He doesn't have a very good bedside manner." That characteristic measures a physician's understanding and application of the art of medicine. Philip Overby says: "Yet the moral virtue of the physician really takes

[72] Hegde BM. Science and the art of medicine, Journal of Indian Academy of Clinical Medicine. 1999;4:1–3.

[73] http://web1.desales.edu/assets/salesian/PDF/GrandRounds.pdf

shape and becomes manifest at the bedside, not in the research laboratory."[74]

A few years back I noticed it seemed quite chic for doctors to make hospital rounds in jeans and tattered short-sleeved shirts—no tie, of course. I was taught differently, and stuck to the dictum given to me as I rounded with the doctors at the hospital where I did my training. Wearing a tie became so ingrained in my routine that I always looked for a reason to wear one, even when I wasn't seeing patients. I have always believed that your personal dress code shows respect to the ones with whom you are working.

About three years ago, I had an experience at the Huntsman Cancer Center in Salt Lake City that reinforced the value of wearing a tie. In the section on Whose In Charge of Your Health I spoke of visiting other doctors' offices as an observer. I called one of the gastroenterologists at the Huntsman Cancer Center and he consented to let me spend half a day with him. The Huntsman is a very attractive facility, besides being one of the most outstanding cancer centers in the U.S., if not the world. As I went down the halls to take my place at the side of one of their gastroenterologists, I was struck by the neat, appropriate dress of every one of the doctors, nurses, and desk folks. They had ties, dress shirts, and nice neat pants or dresses, and most had white lab coats on. I don't remember so much what I learned about medicine that day, but I did learn that the ambience of that center was consistent with their high quality, even to the point of immaculately dressed-up personnel. The stylish dressing-down that I had seen at other places seemed so low class. Yes, looking the part is part of the art of medicine.

The art of medicine is still the foundation of practice, a skill acquired by experience, piggy-backed on an innate caring for people. *Cecil's Textbook of Medicine* states: "The art of caring and comfort, guided by millennia of common sense as well as a more recent systematic approach to medical ethics, remains the cornerstone of medicine. Without these humanistic qualities the application of modern science of 'medicine' is suboptimal, useless, even detrimental."[75]

Diagnosing disease and choosing the best treatment certainly requires scientific knowledge and technical skills in healthcare professionals. For a successful practice, a physician has to be armed with both the science of medicine and the art of medicine. The consummate healers and practitioners of the art of medicine were Dr. Albert Schweitzer and Mother Teresa. And why them? They had a minimum of tools, medicines, and techniques but a maximum of compassion and caring for those they treated.

---

[74] "The Moral Education of Doctors," Phillip J. Overby, *The New Atlantis,* http://www.thenewatlantis.com/publications/the-moral-education-of-doctors
[75] http://www.msmonographs.org/article.asp?issn=0973-1229;year=2006;volume=4;issue=1;spage=127;epage=138;aulast=Panda

# MEDITERRANEAN DIET

The story of man is the story of his great propensity to discover and apply current information, using creativity and cues from his environment. The oldest historic record of these attributes are found in Genesis Chapter 3: 7: "And the eyes of them both were opened, and they knew that they were naked; and they sewed fig leaves together, and made themselves aprons. " This is the simple account of the founding of the clothing industry. Improvements were rapid, for in Genesis Chapter 3: 31, we find them wearing "coats of skin."

Creativity does not necessarily come from just new ideas. I have considered myself creative, but not inventive. As a matter of fact, I can't remember the last time I had a new idea that hadn't already been put forth by someone else. I can't remember the last time I said something that someone, somewhere hadn't already said. Many of the best ideas "shine through" from old ideas. It just takes a good eye to see them, refine them, and make them meaningful to someone who might be interested.

Nothing in this section on the Mediterranean Diet is new. In fact, the Mediterranean Diet was mentioned in the November 5, 2013 issue of *Annals of Internal Medicine*, which looked at a long-term Nurses' Health Study that began in 1976.[76] And nothing in this section comes from my creative abilities. I have merely sorted through the multitude of ideas, suppositions, hypotheses, deductions, and conclusions, then presented them to the reader. You have the greater job of deciding what is relevant, compelling, and worth the time and energy to act upon.

As lifestyle changes begin to firm up, your awareness of self and the environment is the first step.

I think of my one great missed opportunity in life: I could have been the wealthiest man in my neighborhood—or anyone's neighborhood, for that matter. When I was a little boy, I ran through the fields around my dad's nine-acre farm, always returning home with my pants plastered with cockleburs. I pulled them off and threw them away. This "stickiness" characteristic of cockleburs is how Velcro was discovered. Velcro is a combination of the words *velour* and *crochet*. When speaking of Velcro, it's more appropriate to say it was *discovered* rather than *invented*, as nature had been using Velcro since cockleburs plagued Adam and Eve. We just keep finding things that have always been there.

The Mediterranean Diet, too, is not really new. Its inception goes back several decades. The genesis of what we now know as the Mediterranean Diet began with The Seven Countries Study originating in Yugoslavia in 1958.[77] As

---

[76] http://www.reuters.com/article/2013/11/07/us-midlifediet-aging-idUSBRE9A61DR20131107

[77] http://sevencountriesstudy.com/about-the-study/investigators/ancel-keys

one would accurately assume, this study involved seven countries, from the U.S. to Finland. Basically, it told us what many had known almost since the beginning of time—that what we eat has a major bearing on our health.

Since the data of the original study has been analyzed, there has been almost endless research into the diet and implications in the health of not only the U.S. but also the entire world. We in America didn't discover how to prevent and treat cardiovascular disease; we were just smart enough to apply old information into our medical armamentarium.

The most commonly understood version of the Mediterranean Diet was presented by Dr. Walter Willett of Harvard University's School of Public Health in the mid-1990s. Diets which are higher in dietary fruits and vegetables, fish, foods with a large proportion of antioxidant vitamins, flavonoids, and polyphenols result in fewer rates of disease of arteries in various organs. The Mediterranean Diet is the prime example of such a diet and undoubtedly the most extensively studied diet out there. There are hundreds of studies in medicine about the Mediterranean Diet. I will point out only a few which show the positive benefits on our health.

A September 2004 article in *JAMA (Journal of the American Medical Association)* included 1,507 apparently healthy men and 832 women, aged 70 to 90 years, in 11 European countries. This cohort study was conducted between 1988 and 2000. During follow-up, 935 participants died: 371 from cardiovascular diseases, 233 from cancer, and 145 from other causes; for 186, the cause of death was unknown. Adhering to a Mediterranean Diet was associated with a lower risk of all-cause mortality. Similar results were observed for mortality from coronary heart disease, cardiovascular diseases, and cancer. The combination of four low-risk factors lowered the all-cause mortality rate. In total, lack of adherence to this low-risk pattern was associated with a population attributable risk of 60 percent of all deaths, 64 percent of deaths from coronary heart disease, 61 percent from cardiovascular diseases, and 60 percent from cancer. Among individuals aged 70 to 90 years, adherence to a Mediterranean diet and healthful lifestyle was associated with a more than 50 percent lower rate of all-causes and cause-specific mortality.[78] That, my friend, is noteworthy!

**The Basics of the Mediterranean Diet**

Avoid:

1. Snacks and desserts such as cookies, crackers, pretzels, candy bars, cakes, pies, and ice cream contain high amounts of simple carbohydrates.

2. Look out for "hidden sugars" in the guise of ingredients such as brown sugar, molasses, honey, high fructose corn syrup, sorbitol, and juice

---

[78] http://jama.jamanetwork.com/article.aspx?articleid=199485

concentrate.

3. Saturated fat and trans polyunsaturated fats (so-called bad fats). Saturated fat is solid or semi-solid at room temperature and is found predominantly in animal products, with the exception of palm and coconut oils, which are often used in baked goods. Foods containing saturated fat include red meats (beef and lamb), full-fat dairy products, butter, cheese, hot dogs, bacon, sausage, ice cream, and baked desserts. Trans fatty acids are used to lengthen a product's shelf life and are primarily found in stick margarines, fried foods (such as French fries and fried chicken), and processed baked goods (donuts and cakes).

Eat:

1. Monounsaturated fatty acids (MUFAs) and polyunsaturated fatty acids (PUFAs), often called "good fats." Monounsaturated fatty acids (MUFAs) are the preferred dietary fats for patients. The most common monounsaturated fatty acid, oleic acid, is the predominant fatty acid in olives and olive oil. Other dietary sources of MUFA include tree nuts, peanuts, and avocados. New research found that people who ate one-ounce servings of nuts each day had a 20 percent reduction from dying of any cause over three decades, compared to those who didn't eat nuts.

2. Polyunsaturated fatty acids (PUFAs) have also been associated with improved cholesterol profiles. More specifically, PUFAs have been shown to consistently lower fasting triglyceride levels, reducing clotting factors, and improving the health of the endothelium (vessel lining). While most PUFAs are derived from fish, alpha-linolenic acid (ALA), which comes from certain plants, has also been associated with lower cardiovascular risk.

3. Fish, specifically, as your major source of meat. Fish is low in calories and high in omega-3 fatty acids. Choose cold-water fish, including salmon, mackerel, sardines, herring, tuna, and trout. Eat at least two servings of fish per week—grilled or broiled with lemon and herbs rather than fried. Canned tuna is also a popular source of omega-3 fatty acid in the American diet. One six-ounce tin of albacore tuna packed in water contains about a gram of omega-3 fatty acids—approximately a third of the recommended total PUFA. For vegetarians or those who do not like fish, ALA-rich foods such as walnuts, soy, and leeks are good sources of PUFAs. Flaxseeds can be ground into powder and sprinkled onto salads or mixed into cereals and low-fat, low-sugar yogurts.

4. Fiber—Women should aim for 25 grams of fiber per day, while men should

target 38 grams (or 21 and 30 grams daily, respectively, for those over the age of 51). Eating the skin or peel of fruits and vegetables provides a greater dose of fiber, which is found naturally in these sources. Fiber is also found in beans and lentils, whole grains, nuts, and seeds. Typically, the more refined or processed a food becomes, the lower its fiber content.

5. Whole grains are low in fat and are a good source of B vitamins, vitamin E, magnesium, iron, and fiber, as well as other antioxidants. Whole grains release calories into the bloodstream more slowly and improve the cholesterol status of the body. Some of the more common whole grains are: wheat, barley, oats, brown rice, quinoa, rye, millet, and buckwheat.

6. Fruits and Vegetables—It has been well established that eating vegetables and fruits has many health benefits. Most research indicates that it is the antioxidant properties that are responsible for their positive effects. Some of the most widely studied have been ingredients from specific botanical families, including the cabbage family, the lily family (garlic), citrus (such as oranges) and the family that includes tomatoes. At every single meal and snack, choose at least two servings of fruits or vegetables. Some advocates of plant-based diets suggest eating vegetables even between meals, so don't you skip a meal without at least one vegetable serving. At a minimum, eat five to eight servings of fruits or vegetables daily.

BOTTOM LINE: The Mediterranean Diet is the best studied and has the broadest acceptance among researchers and those who understand nutrition.

## THE DASH DIET—DIETARY APPROACHES TO STOP HYPERTENSION

You may be wondering, "Isn't there just one diet that does it all?" Different medical and health organizations and researchers study various diets under a variety of circumstances and clinical protocols. The results indicate that no one diet surpasses all others and that all those folks we look to for answers don't have the same passion for just one diet. You have to decide which is good, better, or best *for you*. Some groups suggest the Mediterranean Diet, others the DASH diet, and still others have data suggesting a plant-based diet is superior.

Nutrition is a key player in combating the environmental influences, which bring about poor health, including high blood pressure. Linda M. Delahanty MS, RD, LDN, chief dietitian and director of nutrition and behavioral research at Massachusetts General Hospital Diabetes Center in Boston, tells us that "nutrition and lifestyle changes can help patients achieve targets for weight loss, glycemic control, blood pressure, and lipid levels with less medication."[79] You undoubtedly picked up on the "less medication." She emphasis what many researchers know: that lifestyle changes can reduce LDL (bad cholesterol) by up to 20 to 30 percent, systolic blood pressure by 19 mm Hg to 50 mm Hg, and diabetes incidence by 58 percent. The reduction of blood pressure mentioned is significant enough to take thousands of people off of blood pressure medication.

Delahanty feels that patents are too often overwhelmed by the number of therapeutic pathways to health, exposed to endless diets and lifestyle changes that "they become so discouraged, frustrated, and confused that they make little to no progress at all. We need to simplify our messages about nutrition and lifestyle, and help patients to prioritize their focus on healthy behaviors."[80] I couldn't agree more, and that is the approach that I encourage. You need an approach that you not only agree with but that is simple enough to follow without excessive coaching.

Focus with me, if you will, on one of the methods used in treating high blood pressure, the DASH diet. The DASH diet has received its widest use and acclaim in the treatment of hypertension (high blood pressure). Hypertension can lead to damaged organs—such as the kidneys, brain (stroke), and heart (heart attack and heart failure)—and dilation of major arteries (aneurysms). Researchers have reported that high blood pressure during middle age may raise the risk of cognitive decline later in life—that means reasoning, memory, etc.

Treatment generally includes changes in lifestyle and medication. The life-

---

[79] http://www.consultant360.com/articles/dietitian-s-perspective-nutrition-cardiometabolic-risk

.[80] http://www.consultant360.com/articles/conference-spotlight-cardiometabolic-risk-summit

style part of the equation is multifactorial, meaning attention needs to be given to appropriate weight loss, dietary intervention, and exercise.

The DASH diet is where the action is, when it comes to dietary treatment of hypertension. DASH stands for *Dietary Approaches to Stop Hypertension*. The DASH diet is a lifelong approach to healthy eating that's designed to help treat or prevent hypertension.

Studies have shown that adherence to this diet, on average, will reduce the systolic blood pressure (the top number) by 11 mm/Hg. Hypertension is the number one chronic disease worldwide. About 70 million adults in the United States have hypertension. According to a report issued by the Centers for Disease Control and Prevention (CDC) in September 2012, over half of all Americans with hypertension do not have their blood pressure under control.[81]

It becomes obvious that diagnosis and treatment are paramount. The DASH diet is rich in fruits, vegetables, grains, and low-fat dairy products, and limits sodium to between 1,500 and 2,300 milligrams a day. The limitation of salt is probably where the diet's power lies. If a person is in wonderful health and all the stats are in that individual's favor, excessive salt intake can still result in increased cardiovascular disease and premature death. We will spend more time on salt intake in another chapter.

Because the DASH diet is a healthy way of eating, it offers health benefits besides just lowering blood pressure. The DASH diet also has a positive impact on prevention of cancer, heart disease, stroke, diabetes, and osteoporosis.

**DASH Diet Specifics**

The table below contains two columns for the number of calories consumed daily—one for 1,600 calories daily, and the other for 2,000 calories daily. Choose the one, which more closely defines the number of calories you eat daily.

| Food Group | Servings for 1,600 Calories/Day | Servings for 2,000 Calories/Day | 1 Serving Example |
|---|---|---|---|
| GRAINS | 6 daily | 6 to 8 daily | • 1 slice whole-wheat bread<br>• 1 oz. dry cereal<br>• ½ cup cooked cereal<br>• ½ cup cooked rice or pasta |

---

[81] http://www.medicalnewstoday.com/articles/150109.php

Whole grains consist of bran, germ, and endosperm—all of the nutrients contained in the original grain seed. Processed grains (i.e. rolled, cracked, crushed, or cooked) are not a good substitute. Whole grains have more fiber. A good rule to follow is to avoid the "five whites": white flour, white pasta, white sugar, white rice, and white potatoes. Whole grains are by nature lower in fat.

However, when buying multi-grain food, be aware that it may not always contain all the grains listed on the package.

Often, seeds and grains are grouped together in this category.

| VEGETABLES | 3 to 4 daily | 4 to 5 daily | • 1 cup raw leafy green vegetables<br>• ½ cup cooked or cut-up vegetables<br>• ½ cup (4 oz.) low-sodium vegetable juice |
|---|---|---|---|

The more colorful the vegetable, the more likely you will maximize your antioxidant intake.

Frozen vegetables are a reasonable alternative when fresh is not possible, with canned as a third choice. When buying frozen or canned vegetables, read labels and choose those without added salt. For the general population, a good rule of thumb is to keep sodium intake to 2,300 mg./day. For those over 50, African Americans, folks with high blood pressure, diabetics, and those with chronic kidney disease, less than 1,500 mg./day.

| FRUITS | 4 daily | 4 to 5 daily | • 1 medium fruit<br>• ¼ cup dried fruit<br>• ½ cup fresh, canned, or frozen<br>• ½ cup (4 oz.) 100% fruit juice |
|---|---|---|---|

Fruits are rich in potassium, magnesium, and fiber and make a great addition to other foods, especially as a snack. To maximize nutritional benefit, eat the skins or peels.

| | | | |
|---|---|---|---|
| DAIRY | 2 to 3 daily | 2 to 3 daily | • 1 cup (8 oz.) milk<br>• 1 cup yogurt<br>• 1 ½ oz. cheese |

Dairy products are a good source of Vitamin D, protein, and calcium. It's ideal to drink low-fat or fat-free milk products, including yogurt. Because cheese contains saturates fats and increased amounts of sodium, it is less beneficial. Almond milk is a good alternative to dairy. It has less calories and more calcium.

| | | | |
|---|---|---|---|
| FISH, POULTRY, AND LEAN MEAT | 3 to 4 or daily | 6 or fewer daily | • 1 oz. cooked lean meat, skinless poultry, or fish<br>• 1 egg (no more than 4 per week)<br>• 2 egg whites |

When choosing meat to eat, go heavy on fish, especially salmon, tuna, herring, mackerel, and sardines, which have the most omega-3. Trim skin away from poultry—that is where the saturated fat is.

| | | | |
|---|---|---|---|
| NUTS, SEEDS AND LEGUMES | 3 to 4 a week | 4 to 5 a week | • 1/3 cup (1.5 oz.) nuts<br>• 2 tbsp. peanut butter<br>• 2 tbsp. (½ oz.) seeds<br>• ½ cup cooked legumes (dried beans or peas) |

Nuts, seeds, and legumes are rich in potassium, magnesium, protein, and phytochemicals, which guard against certain cancers. Though high in calories, nuts contain "good" fatty acids. (There is a chapter on nuts later in this book.)

| | | | |
|---|---|---|---|
| FATS AND OILS | 2 daily | 2 or 3 daily | • 1 tsp. soft margarine<br>• 1 tsp. vegetable oil<br>• 1 tbsp. mayonnaise<br>• 2 tbsp. salad dressing |

The DASH Diet limits total fat to 27 percent of the daily caloric intake. Trans fats are absolutely forbidden, while polyunsaturated and monosaturated fats are encouraged, in the right proportions. Saturated fats should constitute less than 6 percent of total daily caloric consumption. (There is a chapter on Trans fats later in this book.)

| SWEETS AND ADDED SUGARS | 3 or fewer a week | 5 or fewer a week | • 1 tbsp. sugar<br>• 1 tbsp. jelly or jam<br>• ½ cup sorbet<br>• 1 cup (8 oz.) sugar-sweetened lemonade |
|---|---|---|---|

It's always best to avoid sugar whenever possible. Appropriate use of artificial sweeteners such as Splenda, NutraSweet, and Equal can help you consume less white sugar. Note that processed fruit juices are often very high-sugar and should be avoided.

# THE ROLE OF PLANT-BASED DIETS

In the next two chapters we will hear from two of the most awesome experts in the field of plant-based diets. I suggest you buy Dr. Caldwell Esselstyn Jr.'s book *Prevent and Reverse Heart Disease* and T. Colin Campbell's book *The China Study.* Reading them will give you more detail about plant-based diets and the supporting evidence of their efficacy.

Lest you get lost in semantics, the plant-based diet goes by another name: the vegetarian diet. In 2012, about 5 percent of Americans followed a plant-based diet.

The September 7, 2010 issue of *Annals of Internal Medicine* states that a vegetarian diet can meet current recommendations for all necessary nutrients, excepting possibly B12.[82] Noteworthy about plant-based (vegetarian) diets is that they are lower in cholesterol and saturated fat, and higher in fiber, some vitamins and minerals. Vegetarian diets have certain advantages not found in the standard Western diet, such as reduced risk of heart disease, hypertension, lower cholesterol levels and blood pressure, and type 2 diabetes. Vegetarians tend to have lower overall cancer rates. Now that is a real plus!

Well-planned vegetarian diets can be appropriate for individuals during all stages of the lifecycle, including pregnancy, lactation, infancy, childhood, and adolescence, as well as for athletes.

Research has cited the vegetarian diet in the prevention of chronic diseases and the improvement of longevity. Red meat takes a hit when looking into what could possibly be the connection between cardiovascular disease and the foods we eat. In 2012, researchers from the Harvard School of Public Health found that red meat consumption is associated with an increased risk of cardiovascular and cancer death.[83] The same report also showed that there is lower risk of death when there is consumption of healthy protein sources, such as fish, poultry, legumes, and nuts. Investigating the links between disease and different types of diets, Caldwell Esselstyn and Collin Campbell both suggest that a more complete omission of non-plant protein will bring better results. Reading their research, I believe, will convince you that plant-based diets do have merit. These authors' books have a number of recipes and suggestions for making dietary changes.

Chelsea Clinton, the daughter of former President Bill Clinton, said on ABC News about her father, "…his doctor told him that his heart today is much younger than it was even 10 years ago."[84] Since going vegan after his quadruple

---

[82] http://annals.org/article.aspx?articleid=746013

[83] http://www.hsph.harvard.edu/news/press-releases/red-meat-consumption-linked-to-increased-risk-of-total-cardiovascular-and-cancer-mortality/

[84] http://abcnews.go.com/blogs/politics/2014/03/chelsea-clinton-heart-surgery-radically-changed-my-dad/

bypass heart surgery in 2010, Bill Clinton—now 67 years old—"has lost 30 pounds and is feeling better than ever." She also noted that her dad is possibly the world's most famous vegan.

BOTTOM LINE: A plant-based diet has some definite proven advantages over other frequently touted diets, which reduce cardiovascular disease.

# CALDWELL ESSELSTYN'S PLANT-BASED DIET

This is a time for recommitment and a time to become serious about what we are doing. Change needs to occur to bring a better life, a healthier life, and a more productive and purpose-driven life. Are we powerless victims of the winds of the new pervasive immediate self-gratification that embodies our society? Are we caught in the current of secular intellectualism? I hope we can get ourselves off of the reef of entitlement that prevents individual progress. The beacon we must follow is self-awareness and self-determination.

How did we get there? I think at least a part of the answer is the paragraph you just read. This section may hint at the best answer to the question, "What do I need to do to be healthier?" by illustrating where we once were and where we are now.

| DATE | CONSUMED BY EACH PERSON EACH YEAR[85] |
|---|---|
| Turn of the 20th Century | 120 pounds of meat |
| 2007 | 222 pounds of meat |
| 1913 | 40 pounds of processed sugar |
| 2012 | 82 pounds of processed sugar |
| 1909 | 294 pounds of dairy products |
| 2006 | 605 pounds of dairy products |
| Currently | 41.5 pounds of high-fructose corn syrup |
| Currently | 65 pounds fat (2 tons suet by age 60) |

My passion for what goes into the stomach really hit its high point when I read Dr. Caldwell B. Esselstyn's, Jr.'s book *Prevent and Reverse Heart Disease*. Though the numbers of patients Esselstyn studied was small, I felt he was really on to something. He is a very unusual man with unprecedented tenacity in the world of health. To me, his book leaves little doubt that he has advanced the treatment of cardiovascular disease beyond any of his contemporaries. He has an interesting way of portraying his passion: diet.

In an interview with the *Pittsburgh Post-Gazette*, Esselstyn said, "...coronary artery disease and heart attacks are nothing more than a toothless paper tiger that need never, ever exist. If it does exist, it needs never, ever progress. It is a benign food-borne illness. There are multiple cultures on the planet today where if you were to hang out your shingle as a cardiac surgeon—forget it. You'd better

---

[85] http://veggiesforme.com/2011/09/14/shocking-rate-of-increase-of-consumption-of-meat-dairy-and-sugar/

plan on selling pencils. They don't have cardiovascular illness because by culture, heritage and tradition they consume a plant-based diet."[86]

Prevent and Reverse Heart Disease, cover to cover, is 305 pages and contains 150 plant-base recipes. In this chapter, I will extract from his book what I feel would be most helpful and at the same time keep the volume of words down, so that what you will receive will be more palatable. If you want intriguing reading and a boost in your resolve to "enter in at the straight gait" of healthy lifestyle, buy his book. His research is compelling.

First, you need to know Esselstyn's credentials to get a feeling for how real his work and philosophy are and their importance in spelling out what we Americans must do to live to our full health potential. He received an Olympic gold metal in rowing (1956), a bronze star for military service in Vietnam, and was once president of the Cleveland clinic staff. Dr. Esselstyn has been associated with the Cleveland Clinic since 1968. He has been a member of the Board of Governors, Chairman of the Breast Cancer Task Force, head of the Section of Thyroid and Parathyroid Surgery at the Cleveland Clinic, and President of the American Association of Endocrine Surgeons. He has written over 100 professional scientific articles and was chosen in 1994 to 1995 as one of "The Best Doctors in America" by Woodward and White. In 2005, he was the first recipient of the Benjamin Spock Award for Compassion in Medicine.

Esselstyn runs the cardiovascular preventing and reversing program at the Cleveland Clinic Wellness Institute. In 1995, he published the results of his long-term research on arresting and reversing coronary artery disease. That's where you and I come in: his research in arresting and reversing coronary artery disease.

Quoting Dr. Esselstyn:

*All told, there has been little incentive for physicians to study alternate ways to manage disease, so the mechanical, procedural approach continues to dominate the profession even though it offers little to the unsuspecting millions about to become the next victims of disease. Modern hospitals offer almost nothing to enhance public health. They are "cathedrals of sickness." Most all of coronary artery disease is in the Western world. Asia and Africa are in distinct contrast to the 'modern' almost unconscious populous eating whatever their hearts desire, desiring the Golden Arches way of dieting.[87]*

---

[86] http://www.post-gazette.com/ae/breakfast/2013/08/26/Patricia-Sheridan-s-Breakfast-With-Dr-Caldwell-Esselstyn-Jr/stories/201308260142

[87] Prevent and Reverse Heart Disease, Caldwell B. Esselstyn, Jr., M.D., Avery Trade; 1 edition (January 31, 2008)

He continues, "In the United States, where vascular disease is the leading killer, the average citizen eats sixty-five pounds of fat per year—consuming two tons of suet by the age of sixty—and average cholesterol levels hover around 200 mg/dL." For a point of reference, Esselstyn likes to see the total cholesterol level below 150 mg/dL. He uses the phrase *seismic revolution* when talking about plant-based diets. Would it be too bold to suggest that a plant-based diet is the leader in answering the epidemic of cardiovascular deaths?

We now will look at some of the scenarios Dr. Esselstyn points out to reinforce the premise of the superiority of a plant-based diet. These are a few; there are many more.

The Papua Highlanders of New Guinea are traditionally heavy smokers. Their social functions are in communal hutches, so secondhand smoking is part of their culture. The Papua Highlanders suffer many lung disorders as a result of their contact with tobacco. Yet, studies of those who live into their sixties and beyond have shown no coronary artery disease. They are protected by their diet, which consists almost entirely of nineteen separate varieties of sweet potato. Not too appetizing to me, but works for them.

During the Second World War, the Germans occupied Norway and helped themselves to beef and milk—thus the supply for the civilian populous was markedly decreased. Suddenly, Norway was deprived of animal food and dairy. An investigation done by Dr.'s Strom and Jansen analyzed strokes and heart attacks during the war years. During the years 1939 to 1945, deaths from heart attack and stroke "absolutely plummeted." As soon as the Germans left, the cardiovascular diseases returned.

Esselstyn also writes about antioxidants, key in the aging process because they fight free radicals, which accelerate the aging process in our bodies. The body extracts antioxidants from foods, and unfortunately, supplemental antioxidants haven't been shown to be effective in preventing oxidative cellular injury. Esselstyn views eating foods with antioxidants in them (i.e. green leafy vegetables) as medication and suggests one have a couple of vegetable snacks between every meal, just one might take medication for a chronic disease.

What is the mechanism that makes all this happen, or when disease occurs, what is the mechanism that failed? Nitric oxide (NO) dilates vessels and has a number of other important functions, such as producing endothelial relaxation factor, the strongest vasodilator in the body. NO also prevents inflammation in the walls of the vessels. It is found in the one cell layer on the inside of all vessels.

NO declines by 50 percent from the ages of 25 to 50 in the normal aging population, which compromises our cells. Getting older affects us in a number of ways, so we have to maximize the knowledge we have about health. Learn, focus, and apply that which you are learning.

When asked the question "Can a single meal have a negative effect?" Esselstyn answered by referring to the experience of Dr. Vogel of the University of Maryland. Young patients were randomized to a breakfast of cornflakes or hash brown potatoes and sausage. A brachial artery tourniquet was applied, which demonstrates the ability of vessels to dilate. With the tourniquet test, the cuff cuts off systolic pressure on the arm for five minutes. The flow is then measured, the cuff released, and the flow re-measured.

The test demonstrated that bad foods prevent the arteries from full dilation until about 120 minutes after eating. Remember, the ability to respond and dilate quickly is ideal. Think about this: one single meal can prevent arterial dilation. In many of the patients in this experiment, it took them until late afternoon or early evening to recover a nitric oxide response. Those who ate a meal of 900 calories and 50 grams of fat took nearly six hours to dilate. The control group had immediate recovery after release of the tourniquet on the arm.

It can be theorized that each meal could have an accumulative effect on vessels—the vessels you and I depend on for normal brain function, mobility, and response to our environment. This is much like the adverse effects of UVA and UVB rays from the sun in producing skin cancer. Each exposure adds to the total damage. Each sunburn, each overexposure of your skin, produce neoplastic changes that may eventually produce a skin cancer such as melanoma or squamous cell carcinoma. An 800-calorie soggy-with-trans-fat cheeseburger just once a month probably has that sort of accumulative effect on your vessels.

So much is said about the Mediterranean Diet, and rightfully so. It is clearly better than the standard Western diet. However, it's not the best! Dr. Esselstyn maintains that a plant-based diet gives extra coverage beyond what the Mediterranean Diet can provide.

What else about the "holes" in the usual therapy we offer patients? Reported in the *New England Journal:* In a study of several thousand patients, a cholesterol-lowering statin was given. Seventy-five percent of those taking cholesterol-lowering drugs did well in the cardiovascular disease (CVD) category, but the remaining twenty-five percent either sustained a new cardiovascular event or died within a time frame of two and half years.[88] The medical community continues to search for better ways to increase quality of life and longevity.

Though we have a reason to be proud of our advances in medicine, particularly in the cardiovascular realm, we are losing too many people. We think that a procedure can fix anything. I become concerned when I hear patients say, "I can't change my lifestyle; what you see is what you get." When specialists insert stents (to open up coronary arteries) there is a 1 percent mortality rate from

---

[88] *The New England Journal of Medicine*, "Rosuvastatin to Prevent Vascular Events in Men and Women with Elevated C-Reactive Protein," Paul M Ridker, M.D., Eleanor Danielson, M.I.A., Francisco A.H. Fonseca, M.D., Jacques Genest, M.D., Antonio M. Gotto, M.D., John J.P. Kastelein, M.D., Wolfgang Koenig, M.D., Peter Libby, M.D., Alberto J. Lorenzatti, M.D., Jean G. MacFadyen, B.A., Børge G. Nordestgaard, M.D., James Shepherd, M.D., James T. Willerson, M.D., Robert J. Glynn, Sc.D., November 20, 2008 I N Engl J Med 359:2195-2207

the surgery, resulting in 12,000 deaths a year. Four percent of those with stents still have heart attacks.[89] Not bad statistics, but do we have to accept these numbers as "the price of doing business?"

Five hundred thousand bypass surgeries are performed a year[90], with a 3 percent mortality rate[91] — 15,000 deaths a year. Procedures are not without their hazards. There is a better way: healthy lifestyle behavior.

[89] http://www.vegan-magazine.com/2012/07/28/dr-caldwell-esselstyn-discusses-the-problem-with-stents-and-bypass/

[90] http://www.webmd.com/heart-disease/treating-coronary-artery-bypass

[91] http://www.heartprotect.com/mortality-stats.shtml

# PLANT-BASED NUTRITIONAL THERAPY

Dr. Caldwell Esselstyn's recommendations are to avoid all oil, dairy, meat, fish, fowl, sugar, caffeinated coffee, and nuts. (His diet is very critical of any saturated fat—found in nuts, particularly cashews—but nuts are okay if you do not have existing cardiovascular disease.) Instead, consume whole grains, legumes, vegetables, and fruits. Green leafy vegetables should be consumed six times per day because they increase the production of nitric oxide (NO). No olive oil—no oil of any kind. Also, avoid dairy products and anything "with a mother." Fructose (fruit sugar in things like honey, orange juice, and apple juice) is a pox, so avoid it. As for fruits and juices, when you separate the juice from the fiber that is bad, according to Esselstyn, because it changes the glycemic index. Dr. Esselstyn tells his patients that after 12 weeks, they will lose their craving for fat. Conviction and determination are an essential part of your reaching for the stars!

I hope the following chart will give you a good overview of Esselstyn's plant-based diet.[92]

| AVOID | | ALLOWED | |
|---|---|---|---|
| Anything with "a face or a mother" | Meat, poultry, fish, eggs | Vegetables | Sweet potatoes, yams, broccoli, kale, spinach, asparagus, artichokes, eggplant, celery, onions, carrots, Brussels sprouts, corn, cabbage, lettuce, peppers, bok choy, chard, beet greens, squash, tomatoes, cucumbers, etc. |
| Dairy products | Butter, cheese, cream, ice cream, yogurt, milk | Legumes | Beans, peas, lentils |
| Oils | Virgin olive oil, canola oil | Whole grains | Whole wheat, whole rye, bulgur wheat, whole oats, barley, buckwheat, whole corn, cornmeal, wild rice, brown rice, couscous, quinoa, spelt, millet, triticale, faro. |

---

[92] *Prevent and Reverse Heart Disease*, Caldwell B. Esselstyn, Jr., M.D., Avery Trade; 1 edition (January 31, 2008)

| | | | Cereals: shredded wheat, grape nuts |
|---|---|---|---|
| Refined grains | White rice "enriched" flour (bagels, many pastas, baked goods) | Fruit | Fruits of all varieties, but preferably limit fruit to three pieces a day, or for berries, three servings. Avoid pure fruit juices. |
| Nuts | Only with cardiovascular disease, others (may have walnuts) | Beverages | Water, seltzer water, oat milk, no-fat soymilk, coffee, tea |

Those with heart disease should additionally take:
1. Multivitamins
2. Vitamin B12: 1,000 mcg/day
3. Calcium: 1,000 mg/day (over 50 years); 1,200 mg/day (over 60 years)
4. 1,000 I.U./day of Vitamin D (over 50 years)
5. Omega 3 fatty acids, in the form of flaxseed—sprinkle over cereal
6. Statins or other medications as prescribed by your physician

BOTTOM LINE: Buy Dr. Esselstyn's book *Prevent and Reverse Heart Disease.* The closer to a "pure" plant-based diet that you can eat, the better will be your cardiovascular health.

# THE CHINA STUDY

Dr. T. Colin Campbell is an American biochemist and the author of over 300 research papers on nutrition's effects on long-term health. He has written two books: *Whole* (2013) and the book we will focus on, *The China Study* (2005, co-authored with his son). *The China Study* is one of America's best-selling books about nutrition.

In the 1980s, Dr. Campbell was one of the lead scientists of the China Study on diet and disease, created by Cornell University, the University of Oxford, and the Chinese Academy of Preventive Medicine to observe the relationship between nutrition, heart and metabolic diseases, and cancer. It was such a monumental study that the *New York Times* called it "the Grand Prix of epidemiology," and indeed I believe this to be true. This is a book everyone, patient and physician alike, should read.

The research was very expansive. Scientists gathered data on 367 variables and four-dozen diseases, then compared each variable with every other variable. They went into sixty-five counties across China, administered questionnaires, and took blood and urine tests on 6,500 adults. They measured everything families ate over a three-day period and analyzed food samples from marketplaces around the country. The counties were in both rural and semi-rural parts of China. They found that 90 to 94 percent of adults still lived in the same county where they were born—a value-add when drawing final conclusions, because it results in a more homogenous group, which makes results more statistically valid. When they finished their work, they found more than 8,000 significant associations between lifestyle, diet, and disease variables.

Critical to the importance of the China Study was the nature of the diet consumed in rural China. It presented a rare opportunity to study health-related effects of a mostly plant-based diet. The results of the study reinforced the idea that cholesterol blood value is one of the strongest predictors of Western disease—"Western" meaning folks like us who eat the typical disease-producing American diet. It also reaffirmed the notion that as cholesterol decreases, so does cancer, particularly cancers of the liver, colon, lung, and breast. At the time of the study, breast cancer in the U.S. was five times higher than in rural China. The findings in China showed that reducing dietary fat from 24 to 6 percent was associated with lower breast cancer rates.

Coronary artery disease was seventeen times higher in American men than rural Chinese men. That is quite a figure. In an expanded part of their research, the scientists found extraordinarily low rates of coronary heart disease in the southwestern Chinese provinces of Guizhou and Sichuan. During a three-year observation period (1973-1975), there was not one single person who died of coronary heart disease before the age of sixty-four among 246,000 men in

Guizhou County and 181,000 women in Sichuan County. The cholesterol profile of the Chinese participants in these regions was significantly different than their American counterparts. This should get your attention. No single pill or a combinations of pills will give these kinds of results.

Incidentally, Drs. Bill Castelli (longtime director of Framingham Heart Study at NIH), Bill Roberts (editor of the *Journal of Cardiology*), and Caldwell Esselstyn (renowned surgeon at Cleveland Clinic) have never seen a heart disease fatality among their patients who had total blood cholesterol levels below 150mg/dL. Again a powerful statement!

In rural China, animal protein intake averages seven grams a day, while in America, average consumption is a whopping *seventy* grams a day. Animal-based protein increases heart disease; plant protein decreases cholesterol and heart disease. In the U.S., 80 percent of protein consumption is animal protein. This tells quite a story.

We will continue with the checklist under suspicion as culprits in cardiovascular disease. The chart below gives comparisons of the vegetarian and non-vegetarian diets and nutrients in both U.S and Chinese cultures.

**Dietary Comparisons: Vegetarian vs. Non-Vegetarian; China vs. U.S.[93]**

As shown in the chart below, there is only a small difference in the nutritional properties of non-vegetarian and vegetarian diets as consumed in Western countries.

| Vegetarian and Non-vegetarian Diet Comparisons Among Westerners | | |
|---|---|---|
| Nutrient | Vegetarian | Non-vegetarian |
| Fat (% of calories) | 30-36 | 34-38 |
| Cholesterol (g/day) | 150-300 | 300-500 |
| Carbohydrates (% of calories) | 50-55 | < 50 |
| Total protein (% of calories) | 12-14 (10% animal based) | 4-18 |
| Animal protein (% of total protein) | 40-60 | 60-70 |

This next chart shows the marked difference in the various components of a diet consumed by China and the U.S.

| Chinese and American Dietary Intakes | | |
|---|---|---|
| Nutrient | China | United States |
| Calories (kcal/kg body wt/day) | 40.6 | 30.6 |
| Total fat (% of calories) | 14.5 | 34-38 |

[93] *The China Study*, T. Colin Campbell, BenBella Books; 1 edition (May 11, 2006), page 358

| Dietary fiber (g/day) | 33 | 12 |
| --- | --- | --- |
| Total protein (g/day) | 64 | 91 |
| Animal protein (%of total calories) | 0.8 * | 10-11 |
| Total iron (mg/day) | 34 | 18 |

*non-fish animal protein

Lets take a look at fat and carbohydrates.

*The average American dietary style at the beginning of the 21st century resembles an hourglass rather than the Federal Government's Food Guide Pyramid. We gobble up huge amounts of added fats and sugars from the top tier of the pyramid (marked "Use sparingly") and heaping plates of pasta and other refined grains from the bottom tier, but we are sorely lacking in the vegetables, fruits, low-fat milk products, and other nutritious foods in the middle.*
*— http://foodfarmsjobs.org[94]*

In the U.S., we consume 24 percent of our calories in the form of fat.[95] Today, caloric intake by the average American is 3,750 calories a day.[96] That is flat-out too much.

Carbohydrates, our major sources of added sugars, include regular soft drinks, candy, cakes, cookies, pie, fruit drinks, desserts, and milk products such as ice cream, sweetened yogurt, and sweetened milk. According to data from the U.S., in 2008, people consumed over 60 pounds of added sugar per year, not including fruit juices.[97] Fruits, vegetables, and whole grains are the healthiest foods you can consume, and they are primarily made of complex carbohydrates.

The China Study also showed that Chinese fiber intake was three times that of the U.S. The Chinese averaged 30 to 35 grams a day of fiber, and that should be our goal, too. High fiber foods include beans, leafy vegetables, whole fruits, and whole grains.

I've already written about various types of plant-based diets (better know as vegetarian diets). Some are very strict and others leave a little "wiggle room." To recap, a few examples of plant-based diets:

- Vegan (no meat, poultry, fish, dairy, or eggs)
- Vegetarian (no meat, poultry, or fish)

[94] http://foodfarmsjobs.org/wp-content/uploads/2011/09/US-per-Capita-Food-Supply-Trends-More-Calories-Carbs-and-Fat.pdf

[95] http://foodfarmsjobs.org/wp-content/uploads/2011/09/US-per-Capita-Food-Supply-Trends-More-Calories-Carbs-and-Fat.pdf

[96] http://www.fao.org/fileadmin/templates/ess/documents/food_security_statistics/FoodConsumptionNutrients_en.xls

[97] http://ajcn.nutrition.org/content/94/3/726.full

- Pesco-vegetarian (no meat or poultry, but fish allowed)
- Semi-vegetarian (red meat less than once a month, and poultry less than once a week)

# DIETARY PROTEIN

To understand the link between protein source and mortality, the journal *Cell Metabolism* reported on a study of caloric restriction (without malnutrition). The question that was posed: "Is animal protein bad for your health?" The long answer: Middle-aged people who eat lots of animal protein are four times more likely to die of cancer.[98]

The study, conducted by U.S. and Italian researchers, followed thousands of adults for nearly two decades as they consumed animal protein derived from lots of meat, milk, and cheese.

In a *Washington Post* article about the study, Valter Longo, a University of Southern California gerontology professor and director of the school's Longevity Institute, states, "The great majority of Americans could reduce their protein intake. The best change would be to lower the daily intake of all proteins, but especially animal-derived proteins."[99]

A high protein diet is one that has 20 percent or more of its daily caloric intake in protein. A low-protein diet is defined as having less than 10 percent of daily calories in protein. The study, factoring in educational, health, and ethnic backgrounds, also points out that eating lesser amounts of protein, but still staying above the recommended amount, over time, still has a deleterious effect.

Longo also points out that the problem with the middle-aged, high protein consumption group is a worldwide challenge. "People are eating twice and sometimes three times as much protein as they need, with too much of that coming from animals rather than plant-based foods such as nuts, seeds, and beans."[100]

Longo's recommendation is that middle-aged adults should not exceed the recommended intake of 0.8 grams of protein per kilogram of body weight daily. He suggests following the example of the folks in the small, southern Italian town of Molochilo, which has one of the highest rates of centenarians in the world. A large number of villagers maintain a low-protein, plant-based diet. These dietary habits are not new to many around the world. Plant-based diets have proven to be superior to our standard Western diet of eating just about anything our hearts desire without regard to consequences.

Dr. Robert A. Vogel, a cardiologist at the University of Colorado, at Denver, says, "If I had one recommendation based upon all the data I've reviewed, it would be to become a pesco-vegetarian. They in fact are the longest-

---

[98] http://www.cell.com/cell-metabolism/fulltext/S1550-4131(14)00062-X

[99] http://www.washingtonpost.com/national/health-science/too-much-protein-could-lead-to-early-death-study-says/2014/03/04/0af0603e-a3b5-11e3-8466-d34c451760b9_story.html

[100] http://www.washingtonpost.com/national/health-science/too-much-protein-could-lead-to-early-death-study-says/2014/03/04/0af0603e-a3b5-11e3-8466-d34c451760b9_story.html

living Americans. Seventh-day Adventists as a group have the longest life expectancy among all Americans."[101] (A pesco-vegetarian is a vegetarian who also consumes fish and seafood.)

The Adventist Health Study-2 was conducted over 5.8 years and reported on 73,308 participating Seventh-day Adventists from both the U.S. and Canada. The diets they ate varied. The risk of all-cause mortality (death from any cause) was 12 percent lower among vegetarians than non-vegetarians, and 19 percent lower in the pesco-vegetarian group. Also within the group, 8 percent were vegans (not eating any animal products); 29 percent were lacto-ovo-vegetarians (not eating fish or meat, but eating dairy and egg products); 15 percent occasionally ate meat, including fish.

The investigators concluded that less-than-once-weekly meat consumption was a major factor accounting for increased longevity in these people. Very low meat intake resulted in a significant prolongation of life—an additional. 3.6 years.

The Nurses' Health Study and Health Professionals Follow-Up Study, which studied the eating habits of120,000 men and women, carried on for more than two decades and showed that "those who ate the most red meat tended to die younger from cardiovascular disease and cancer, even after the researchers compensated for the effects of smoking, being overweight, and other unhealthy lifestyle influences."[102]

Even smaller amounts of processed food increase the death rate from cardiovascular disease. "Consuming less than half a serving (1.5 ounces) per day of red meat could have prevented about one in 10 premature deaths in men in the study." [103]

BOTTOM LINE: Young or old, cutting down on animal protein lessens the likelihood of dying from metabolic diseases and cancer. Focus on plant-based proteins, such as beans, nuts, and seeds. Vegetarians may not be so misdirected after all!

---

[101] http://www.practiceupdate.com/news/4318

[102] http://www.health.harvard.edu/press_releases/sins-of-the-flesh-if-meat-isnt-so-good-for-you-how-do-you-get-healthy-protein

[103] http://www.health.harvard.edu/press_releases/sins-of-the-flesh-if-meat-isnt-so-good-for-you-how-do-you-get-healthy-protein

# ORNISH DIET

Dr. Dean Ornish began his medical training at the Baylor College of Medicine and later became a Clinical Fellow in Medicine at Harvard Medical School. He is the author of many best-selling books, including *Dr. Dean Ornish's Program for Reversing Heart Disease*; *Eat More, Weigh Less*; *Love & Survival*; and his most recent book, *The Spectrum*. Our look into his life and work will be about his diet.

Dr. Ornish's training put him in a good position to establish a brilliant medical career. He is probably best known for his study the Lifestyle Heart Trial. The subjects had pre-existing coronary artery disease, and the treatment of those patients was based on lifestyle changes, which included a whole foods, plant-based diet, moderate exercise, smoking cessation, stress management techniques including yoga and meditation, and psychosocial support on preventive health. About 48 patients enrolled in the study. After one year of treatment, of those who had experienced chest pain in the past, 65 percent had eliminated their chest pain.

Overall, 82 percent of the experimental-group patients had an average change toward regression of their coronary artery disease. After three years, 60 percent had no chest pain. Average total cholesterol starting level was 227 mg/dL and went down to 172 mg/dL, and the LDL dropped from 152 mg/dL to 95 mg/dL. Those are significant changes for the better.[104]

Those with his dietary regimen did better with respect to coronary events and additionally showed regression of the coronary atherosclerosis (hardening of the arteries), prompting the question: Why are so many procedures such as artery bypass surgery and stents performed?

In 2010, after President Bill Clinton's bypass vessels became plugged, Dr. Ornish encouraged him to follow a more rigid plant-based diet, because previous moderate dietary changes had not stopped the progression of the president's coronary artery disease. The results of this intervention have proven to be effective.

After publication of his research, Dr. Ornish negotiated with an insurance company to try his program on patients scheduled for bypass surgery. The results were exceptional: it was estimated that the insurance company saved about $30,000 per patient. [105] Eventually, more and more insurance companies were convinced. Finally, in 2010, Medicare started covering the Dean Ornish Program for rehabilitation of heart patients. This underlines the sound basis for

---

[104] http://www.ornishspectrum.com/wp-content/uploads/Intensive-lifestyle-changes-for-reversal-of-coronary-heart-disease1.pdf

[105] http://www.positivehealth.com/article/clinical-practice/efficacy-of-lifestyle-intervention-programmes-in-the-treatment-of-non-communicable-lifestyle-related

plant-based therapy.

One of the positive points of the Ornish Diet is the ability to make different choices, depending upon your personal goals. Freedom of choice is a cornerstone of his dietary therapy. A motivated person can select a diet with major changes, or select something they think is more doable.

## Ornish Diet Details[106]

The Ornish diet focus is more on what you eat, and not so much on calorie consumption. Instead of counting calories, Ornish says that when you're hungry, you should eat until you are full. Of course, "eat until you are full" is open to wide interpretation. Certainly it has something to do with being satisfied, not stuffed.

He describes three categories: foods that should be eaten all of the time, some of the time, and none of the time. Sounds pretty simple.

EAT ALL OF THE TIME
> Beans and legumes
> Fruits
> Grains
> Vegetables

EAT IN MODERATION
> Nonfat dairy products—skim milk, nonfat yogurt, nonfat cheeses, nonfat sour cream, and egg whites. I hope you are getting the picture: avoid foods with saturated fats.
>
> Nonfat or very low-fat commercially available products—from Life Choice frozen dinners to Haagen-Dazs frozen yogurt bars and Entenmann's fat-free desserts. But if sugar is among the first few ingredients listed, avoid it.

FOODS TO AVOID
> Meat of all kinds—red and white, fish and fowl (if you can't give up meat, at least eat as little as possible, with fish being the best choice). This is more in line with the vegetarian diet, a diet proven to be very beneficial to health.
> Oils and oil-containing products, such as margarine and most salad dressings (no olive or canola oil)
> Avocados
> Olives
> Nuts and seeds

---

[106] http://ornishspectrum.com

Dairy products (other than the nonfat ones above)
Sugar and simple sugar derivatives—honey, molasses, corn syrup, high-fructose syrup
Alcohol
Anything commercially prepared that has more than two grams of fat per serving

If you stick to this diet, you will consume less than 10 percent of your calories from fat, without the need to count fat grams or calories.

Dr. Ornish also recommends additional lifestyle changes including stress management activities, such as meditation and relaxation, and exercising a minimum of three hours a week.

BOTTOM LINE: The Ornish Diet is a more user-friendly diet which looks a lot like a vegetarian diet. It has proven significant cardiovascular benefits.

# OKINAWA DIET

In 2001, *The Okinawa Program*, written by Dr. Brad Willcox, was a New York Times Bestseller and was nominated as Best Wellness Book of the Year by the Multiple Sclerosis Society[107], so it's an important diet to mention. Like many diets, over a period of time, the initial hype tends to die down, but the research and resultant dietary suggestions still have merit.

Okinawans seem to have better health and longevity than other Japanese and Americans, in part due to decreased incidence of heart disease, stroke, and cancer. Centenarians number about 34 per 100,000 people, compared with 5 to 10 centenarians per 100,000 in America.

The average Okinawan is eight times less likely to die from coronary heart disease, seven times less likely to die from prostate cancer, six and a half times less likely to die from breast cancer, and two and a half times less likely to die from colon cancer than the average American. Of equal importance, Okinawans have an eight- to nine-year longer lifespan, and at the end of life, live with less disability and loss of function.

The study showed that inhabitants of the island of Okinawa ate 30 percent fewer calories and had a 35 percent lower rate of cardiovascular disease and cancer mortality than the average Japanese population. What might the answer be for this remarkable statistic? Diet, exercise, stress management, and social interaction — especially with family and spirituality — seem to be the factors responsible for the health of this culture. [108]

Lets have a look into the dietary habits of the Okinawans and examine how we can incorporate their lifestyle into our own health behavior.

Okinawan elders eat, on average, seven to ten servings of vegetables and fruit, seven servings of grain, and two servings of soy products each day. The older, healthier elders also eat a great deal of sweet potatoes. However, over the last several years, dietary practices in Okinawa have been shifting toward Western and mainstream Japanese patterns, with fat intake rising from about 10 to 27 percent of total caloric intake, and the sweet potato being steadily supplanted with rice and bread. The older group of Okinawans eat fish (rich in omega-3) several times a week, minimal dairy products, and about an ounce of poultry or pork daily. Fish is certainly a better choice of meat than chicken or pork. Pork should be way down on the list of meats. Okinawa's indigenous vegetables include purple sweet potatoes rich in flavonoids, carotenoids, vitamin E, and lycopene; the local bitter cucumbers, or *goya*, have been shown to lower blood sugar in those with diabetes.

---

[107] http://orcls.org/bradley_willcox.php

[108] *The Okinawa Program : How the World's Longest-Lived People Achieve Everlasting Health--And How You Can Too*, Bradley J. Wilcox, Harmony (March 12, 2002)

How do Okinawans cook their food? They typically fry at a low temperature, using canola oil, which is very low in saturated fat and high in monounsaturated fatty acids, which reduces LDL and raises HDL. However, canola oil and olive oil are very similar, so if you prefer olive oil, that is okay. My educated preference is canola oil.

Okinawan elders strive to stop eating before they're full—very different than the average American. Okinawans call this strategy *hara hachi bu,* which means, "Eat until you are eight parts full." (Eight out of ten, that is.) But the feeling of fullness is very subjective, and this practice is open for considerable speculation—how do you measure 80 percent full?

When Okinawans leave the island and abandon their traditional ways, they tend to reap the consequences of lifestyle changes, and as the Western world creeps in to Okinawa, effects are being seen. "On Okinawa, the prevalence of fast-food restaurants and convenience stores that purvey snacks no doubt will exact a toll on the health of younger Okinawans who patronize them," says Dr. Bradley Willcox, a Mayo Clinic-trained internist and a geriatrics fellow in Harvard University's Division on Aging, who participated in the study.[109]

Dr. Willcox also says, "There are over 100,000 Okinawans in Brazil. They eat 18 times more meat, almost double the processed meat, 3.4 times as much sugar, 2.5 times as much milk products, 1.2 times more salt, and only 70 percent of the fish and vegetables that Okinawans on Okinawa eat."[110] He observes that the number of centenarians in Brazil is only one-fifth that in Okinawa.

In addition to their eating habits, older Okinawans have a deep spirituality, are involved in worship, and are religious leaders of society. Socialization and family are an integral part of their daily living. A lot of them belong to community centers.

And regarding their diet, which is of course the key: they eat plant-based foods, green and yellow vegetables, whole grains, legumes, tofu, fish, and especially soy. They consume minimal amounts of sugar, very little meat, and very little dairy or eggs. Their diet is high in complex carbohydrates. They do have an occasional alcoholic drink. For more information, conduct an online search on "Okinawa Diet Food Pyramid." It very accurately depicts the foods they eat, along with the number of servings.

BOTTOM LINE: Eat low-glycemic index foods (less simple carbohydrates) and less caloric-dense foods. Concentrate more on plant-based foods, with ten servings of fruits and vegetables daily. Obtain and maintain appropriate weight.

---

[109] http://www.okicent.org/news/chicago_tribune.html

[110] http://articles.chicagotribune.com/2001-06-24/news/0106240441_1_okinawans-centenarians-okinawa-program/2

# THE COLOR CODE DIET AND ANTIOXIDANTS

The book *The Color Code* is about colored fruits and vegetables, and contains The Color Code Eating Program. Colorful, fresh produce is one of the keys of any diet to obtain optimal health. The prime movers in fruit and vegetables—the substances most beneficial for good health—are the antioxidants.

A few examples of color and benefits:

1. The red (lycopene) in red tomatoes can cut the incidence of prostate cancer in half.
2. The red in cherries helps lessen the symptoms of arthritis.
3. The yellow in corn helps with retinal health.
4. The beautiful indigo in blueberries help the aging brain.
5. Phytochemicals found in fruits and vegetables help fight off cancer.

Plants, in order to protect their protoplasm from ultraviolet light, have pigments lessening the harmful effects of solar irradiation. When we eat these plants, we mobilize those components to protect our bodies, muting the inflammatory process, which is inevitable in each one of us.

The normal metabolic process causes oxidation. The byproduct of this normal chemical reaction is free radicals. Environmental factors, pollution, cigarette smoke, and sun exposure are other causes of free radical production. Free radicals damage DNA and parts of the body's cells, and contribute to the aging process as well as diseases such as diabetes, cancer, and heart disease. And it is believed that oxidation plays a role in the development of fatty deposits in the walls of blood vessels, which increases the risk of heart attack and stroke.

Antioxidants are natural substances that limit the damage produced by free radicals. Your body uses antioxidants to stabilize those free radicals. Appropriate food choices will supply you with all the antioxidants necessary to maintain optimal health. Because there are a variety of antioxidants going about doing their various types of good deeds, it is important to eat different fruits and vegetables, rather than just concentrating on one food.

There is very little evidence, by the way, that taking supplements can replace or maintain antioxidants you get by eating a variety of vegetables and fruits.

So what foods are good sources of antioxidants and what are some antioxidants?

Vitamin A is found in fortified oatmeal, fortified skim milk (non-fat), peaches, tomatoes, green peas, and mangoes. Vitamin C is found in broccoli, Brussels sprouts, cauliflower, papayas, strawberries, oranges, cantaloupe, bell peppers, tomatoes, and kale. Vitamin E is found in some nuts and seeds, including almonds, hazelnuts, and peanuts. Other sources of vitamin E are green leafy vegetables and oils, such as soybean and canola oils.

Beta-carotene is found in cantaloupe, apricots, mangoes, peaches, broccoli, carrots, peas sweet potatoes, squash, spinach, and kale. Lutein is found in broccoli, spinach, corn, orange pepper, kiwi fruit, grapes, zucchini, squash, and kale. Lycopene is found in pink and red fruits and vegetables, such as pink grapefruit, watermelon, apricots, and tomatoes. Selenium is found in cereals (corn, wheat, and rice), nuts, legumes, animal products (beef, fish, turkey, chicken, and eggs), bread, and pasta.

Note: Maybe someone is looking to the future. The USDA's Natural Resources Conservation Service recently released The National Resources Inventory, which shows an increase in land dedicated to growing fruits, nuts, and flowers—from 124,800 acres in 2007 to 273,800 in 2010.[111]

Choosing whole fruits is very important. We know that greater consumption of specific whole fruits, particularly blueberries, apples, and grapes, is definitely associated with a lower risk of type 2 diabetes, whereas increased consumption of fruit juices has the opposite association. There is more than one reason for this, but we know that higher intake of fructose is injurious to health. Getting your juice with your fiber by eating whole fruits is a better deal.

The two major contributors to the book The Color Code are James Joseph, M.D. and Daniel A. Nadeau, M.D. Dr. Nadeau is Medical Director of the Health Reach Diabetes, Endocrine, and Nutrition Center and Assistant Professor of Medicine at Tufts Medical School in Boston. According to Nadeau, "If we can reduce the inflammation in our bodies by eating fruits and vegetables, we are not only protecting ourselves from these conditions, but we are protecting ourselves from aging itself."[112]

Dr. Joseph was head of the USDA-ARS Human Nutrition Research Center on Aging (HNRCA) at Tufts University as the director of the Neuroscience Laboratory until his death in 2010. His studies with blueberries and rodents earned him the title of "The Blueberry King." Dr. Joseph's contributions have earned him, among other awards, the Stephanie Overstreet Award in Alzheimer Research.

There are varying opinions on how many servings of fruits and vegetables you should eat daily. The USDA suggests a total of five to nine servings a day— that is, three to five servings of vegetables and an additional two to four servings of fruit. The DASH diet, originally constructed to help treat high blood pressure, prescribes 10 servings of fruits and vegetables a day.

**Weight loss advantages:** Fruits and vegetables are not calorie-dense. For example, a cup of blueberries contains only 80 calories. To consume 2,000 calories in a day—about the average daily caloric consumption—you would have to eat 25 cups of blueberries. By increasing fruits and vegetables in your diet, you

---

[111] http://blogs.usda.gov/2014/01/23/report-cultivated-fruit-nut-and-flower-acres-on-the-rise/

[112] http://www.wildblueberryhealthblog.com/2012_07_01_archive.html

will naturally cut down on white foods such as white rice, white flour in any form, white potatoes, and white pasta.

Of course, a semi-vegetarian diet is a good choice for good health and weight reduction.

# SMELL: WHAT THE NOSE KNOWS

Much of the pleasure of food and our motivation to eat lies in the flavor, taste, and smell of food. Smell is a sense whose value seems to be only really appreciated after it is lost. The disease characterized by loss of smell is called *anosmia*.

Anosmia is an inability to detect odors and can cause significant physical and social maladies. The first recorded scientific observations of anosmia were made by Hughling Jackson in 1864, who wrote, "In 1837 a gentleman of Sheepwash in Devon was struck from his horse. All the worst effects of concussion resulted—his sense of smell was lost forever."[113]

Anosmic patients can experience problems related to their food intake with either excessive weight gain or loss. Anosmic people forced to rely solely upon their sense of taste—sweet, salty, bitter, and sour—are truly in a position to appreciate the actual value of the sense of smell in the eating process.

Your sense of smell—and the way your food looks—initiates chemosensory signals that prepare the body to ingest food by triggering salivary, gastric, pancreatic, and intestinal secretions. These senses enable us to detect and discriminate among foods that are nutritious as well as pleasant to consume. Learned associations between a food's taste and smell and its post-ingestive effects enable us to monitor and change food intake in anticipation of its nutritional benefits, or for that matter, its deleterious effects on health. The ability to smell is a guidepost to proper food consumption. Likewise, taste and smell signals initiate, sustain, and encourage termination of food ingestion—critical whether you are thin, fat, or "just right."

The response to smell is learned over a lifetime and incorporated into our eating habits early on in our lives. Of course, that which smells good may often be less healthful than that which does not turn you on in an olfactory sense. Good judgment must therefore override what you have learned, such as the delicious smell of meat, potatoes, and gravy—foods many of us grew up eating. Meat, potatoes, and gravy are secondary to nothing else in life. There is nothing so exciting and ultimately rewarding than that first forkful!

## Smell as a Tool to Determine Disease

Approximately 5.2 million Americans have Alzheimer's or another form of dementia, according to the Alzheimer's Association, with about 13.8 million cases expected by 2050. Creative researchers at the University of Florida's McKnight

---

[113] http://chemse.oxfordjournals.org/content/24/6/705.full

Brain Institute Center for Smell and Taste have provided us with some very interesting information about our "smeller." Their pilot study, centered around Alzheimer's disease, was published in a recent issue of the *Journal of Neurological Sciences.*[114]

Alzheimer's disease affects many areas of the brain, but most often begins in the olfactory area, the smelling portion. The University of Florida study showed that Alzheimer's patients have more difficulty smelling peanut butter held at a specified distance from their nose than those without the disease.[115] The olfactory area of the brain may be affected even before the decline in memory occurs.

You can test yourself with the help of an assistant. The testing goes something like this: Take a tablespoon of peanut butter and a metric ruler, close your eyes and mouth, and block one nostril. Move the peanut butter container one centimeter at a time up the ruler until you can detect the odor. (Remember to use a metric ruler, or do the math: one inch equals 2.54 centimeters.) Ninety seconds later, repeat the test with the other nostril. The test is considered positive if you find that you need to be 10 centimeters or less closer on the left nostril than the right to first smell the peanut butter.

BOTTOM LINE: While you are counting your blessings, add to the list your ability to smell life's various odors and fragrances.

---

[114] http://www.alz.org/alzheimers_disease_facts_and_figures.asp
[115] http://news.ufl.edu/archive/2013/10/uf-researchers-find-that-peanut-butter-test-can-help-diagnose-alzheimers-disease.html

# ANTIOXIDANT COMPARISON

Trolox is a water-soluble antioxidant compound similar to vitamin E—a "scavenger" in the brain, designed to help clean up oxidized substances and byproducts produced by brain tissue. Oxidation, remember, contributes to aging and deteriorating brain function. Trolox works by picking up the extra electrons from the oxidation process.

Trolox is certainly not the only substance neuro-research is interested in, but the following chart will give you an idea of what foods have the best chance of maximizing this "cleaning" method the brain has. The higher the number, the better. They are listed in equivalent/gram.[116]

| FRESH FRUIT | | VEGGIES AND LEGUMES | |
|---|---|---|---|
| Blueberries | 2400 | Kale | 1700 |
| Blackberries | 2036 | Spinach | 1260 |
| Cranberries | 1750 | Brussels sprouts | 980 |
| Strawberries | 1540 | Alfalfa sprouts | 930 |
| Raspberries | 1220 | Broccoli | 890 |
| Plums | 949 | Beets | 840 |
| Avocadoes | 782 | Red bell peppers | 460 |

When you have a choice, go for the fruits and vegetables closer to the top. Include these in your daily diet.

Color gives you an idea of what is in a type of food. With a broad sweep of the brush, let me give you the "color" method for finding antioxidants.

**Orange**
Oranges (vitamin C)
Carrots (beta-carotene)
Sweet potatoes/yams (beta-carotene)

**Red**
Tomatoes (vitamin C, lycopene)
Apples (quercetin)

**Blue**
Blueberries (flavonoids, anthocyanin, vitamin E)

---

[116] http://www.doterra-aromatics.com/info/orac.html

**Green**

Broccoli (indole-3-carbinol, sulforaphane)
Asparagus (folate, B vitamins, glutathione)
Spinach (beta-carotene, lutein, flavonoids)

Another very important point to remember is that no combination or amount of supplements can provide the same value as eating a healthy, varied diet. Of course, this becomes more and more difficult to do as we get older and we begin to lose our sense of taste and our appetite changes. Though fresh vegetables and fruit are always best, not everyone can get to the store every day. Frozen ones are okay, too. For people with restricted diets by necessity, the correct supplements are a good second choice.

BOTTOM LINE: Eat an abundance of fruits and vegetables from each color group every day. Try to make blueberries a regular item in your diet.

# TAKE A BREAK

Maybe this would be a good time to get off of the healthy lifestyle treadmill and have a good look at where you are, in terms of your health. When you have your breath back, you can resume your quest for a more healthy future. Remember, "If it is going to be, it's up to me."

My experience tells me that as much as people want to change their behavior, it can be very difficult to do. Sometimes it seems there is so little improvement after so many sunrises. I have asked, and will continue to ask you, to change your behavior. This is your time to stop and analyze where you are and ask the question, "Am I headed in the right direction?" I want you to stop, reset the sail, recalculate the course, fine tune, reexamine, and see where and why you are at this point in your quest for healthy lifestyle changes.

For a little boost to reignite your resolve, look again at your purpose in life. Ask yourself, "Have I delivered the message that I need to deliver to mankind?" Or, as I once heard asked so wisely, "Have I played the music in me?"

"Each day is a separate life, and each evening is a time to review it," said Pythagoras. Certainly, reviewing the events of each day, at the end of the day, is important in pursuit of your goals. However, without the foundation of commitment, an evening review is like watering rows where you didn't plant seeds. Reviewing the day's events at day's end only has value if there is fundamental determination to change and make tomorrow a day of labor and change.

Your next question should be, "Am I willing to devote the effort it takes to reach my goals?" Changing behavior is so much about changing habits. By now, you have developed some good habits, which act as stepping-stones to your ultimate success.

Your motivation—how badly you want to change—is perhaps the key to changing behavior, and what you are willing to give up or do to make that change is what personal motivation is all about. I have given you a great deal of information to help you take the right steps, hopefully without making you feel guilty or causing fear in your heart. As we have been moving along, I hope I have gotten into your heart as well as into your head. At the beginning of the book I spoke of trust and the importance of developing the "in your heart" partner relationship. Believe in what we are doing together! Belief creates a willingness to try. Trying with faith in yourself and undaunted effort will bring about success.

As we have already discussed, leaving the past behind you has been a valuable move. Discarding that which is baggage and that which is counterproductive to your success is a good move. Pat yourself on the back, and let's move forward. Be gentle with yourself, but maintain a wholesome discipline.

The miracle of modern medicine and the expertise provided by the many and varied caregivers we have access to add, on average, three to seven years of life per person. But individually, and as a nation, we can do better. We will do better, but we need a new direction.

The year I started my medical practice, 1960, the GDP (gross domestic product) was 6 percent. Now it is nearly 18 percent, and climbing. GDP is the market value of all officially recognized final goods and services produced within a country in a year or other given period of time. GDP-per-capita is often considered an indicator of a country's standard of living.

The Affordable Care Act is the current American fix for our health problems. It is far from the health reform that we are so badly in need of—it is an insurance fix, not a heath reform. So, let us step in and do what our government, bless their hearts, thinks they are doing for us. We have an opportunity. On BYUTV in March, 2014, Brent James talked about the opportunity that is ahead of us. He began by pointing out our nation's healthcare deficiencies. Here is the list.[117]

1. Well-documented, massive variation in practice beyond the level where it is even remotely possible that all patients are receiving good care
2. High rates of inappropriate care
3. Unacceptable rates of preventable care associated with patient injury and death
4. A striking inability to "do what we know works"
5. A huge amount of waste, leading to spiraling prices that limit access to medical care (46.6 million uninsured people); fifty percent of all resource expenditure is quality-associated waste—including inefficiency and the providing of unnecessary treatments

The figures and information in this section were obtained from "National Debt Facts" by James D. Agresti. I suggest for your edification you go online and reference his article. He has details that are well researched and come from many sources. With the information below in mind, I will explain why I feel you need to be aware of these facts.

Currently, the official debt of the United States government is $17.6 trillion. This amounts to:

- $55,419 for every person living in the U.S.
- $143,976 for every household in the U.S.
- 102 percent of the U.S. gross domestic product

---

[117] http://www.byutv.org/watch/0d7cb22d-1592-49ec-81a7-e1f636f959b8/byu-forum-address-brent-james-31814

- 540 percent of annual federal revenues[118]

Now, here is where it gets interesting. The following figures are called "shortfalls." As of September 30, 2013, the federal government had roughly:

- $7.8 trillion in liabilities that are not accounted for in the national debt
- $23.8 trillion in obligations for current Social Security participants above and beyond projected revenues from their payroll and benefit taxes
- $27.3 trillion in obligations for current Medicare participants above and beyond projected revenues from their payroll taxes, benefit taxes, premium payments, and assets of the Medicare trust fund[119]

Get out your pencil and paper and do a little math. Put in the equation shortfalls plus the national debt, then subtract the value of federal assets, and you'll come up with the federal government owing about $71 trillion in debts, liabilities, and unfinanced obligations. If you can stop your head from spinning for a moment, read this: This shortfall is 92 percent of the combined net worth of all U.S. households and nonprofit organizations, including all assets in savings, real estate, corporate stocks, private businesses, and consumer durable goods such as automobiles. This includes our homes, furniture, clothes, groceries, etc.

Now, let's look at a new set of figures. This shortfall alone equates to:
- $224,110 for every person living in the U.S.
- $579,761 for every household in the U.S.
- 420 percent of the U.S. gross domestic product[120]

Why do I feel this information is important to you? You need to know that currently 38.7 trillion of the shortfall is from Medicare. Medicare is our country's national social insurance program. It guarantees access to health insurance for Americans aged 65 and older who have worked and paid into the system, and younger people with disabilities as well as people with end-stage renal disease and persons with amyotrophic lateral sclerosis. The Medicare shortfall is the difference between the money the program brings in and the money it spends on healthcare benefits. The Heritage Foundation tells us that even assuming that unrealistic cost-containment policies in current law are sustained, by 2040, Medicare's shortfall will account for 81 percent of the federal deficit.

Addressing runaway federal deficits requires targeting Medicare. If you are not using Medicare at this point, somewhere down the line, you probably will have that opportunity. Medicare's 2013 annual report tells us that the program's

[118] http://www.justfacts.com/nationaldebt.asp
[119] http://www.justfacts.com/nationaldebt.asp
[120] http://www.justfacts.com/nationaldebt.asp

financial projections "do not represent a reasonable expectation for actual program operations in either the short range … or the long range."

So, if you are relying on Medicare to take care of you, depending on how quickly we run out of other people's money, it will not be your safety net. I am certain Medicare will not go away, but it will change significantly.

In their retirement years, my parents weren't wealthy by any means, but I thought they could take care of themselves pretty well. When Medicare was enacted in 1966, I remember my mother talking about getting on it. She had been paying her medical bills out of pocket and from my father's teacher's insurance program. My immediate reaction was, "Not my folks, no way are they going on government subsidy!" Of course, after the initial "sticker shock" of Medicare, not only were my parents being parented by our government, but I became the government's "in the trenches" medical representative as a family practitioner. Government in our lives is a way of life now.

Still, as our own practitioners, we can do better for ourselves than that.

An American reporter had the opportunity to visit the Schweitzer Clinic in Lambaréné, Gabon. The day after arriving at the clinic, Dr. Schweitzer took the reporter to watch the witchdoctors work. The reporter had worried Dr. Schweitzer with a comment a day earlier: "These local people are very lucky to have access to the Schweitzer Clinic instead of having to depend upon witch doctor supernaturalism."

As scheduled, the group took off to watch the witchdoctors at work. With some patients, the witch doctor merely put herbs in a brown bag and instructed as to their use. With other patients, he gave no herbs but instead filled the air with incantations. A third category of patients he merely spoke to in a subdued voice and pointed to Dr. Schweitzer.

Dr. Schweitzer could tell the reporter didn't quite have it all figured out, so he explained the first group would improve very rapidly, since they had only functional rather than real organic disease disturbances. The second group had psychological ailments that were being treated with African psychotherapy. The third group had more substantial physical problems such as hernias, dislocated joints, tumors, and so forth. Many of these problems required surgery, and the witch doctor was redirecting the patients to Dr. Schweitzer.

Dr. Schweitzer said, "Some of my steadiest customers are referred to me by witch doctors. Don't expect me to be too critical of them." Then, the American reporter was told the essence of medical therapy. "The witch doctor succeeds for the same reason all the rest of us succeed. Each patient carries his own doctor inside him. They come to us not knowing the truth. We are at our best when we give the doctor who resides within each patient the chance to go to work."

This took place about a century ago, and the message is still the same: we give the doctor who resides within each patient the chance to go work. When the patient understands this concept of control of self, then that patient knows he must direct his own life. Being a purveyor of the truth, the physician can be an essential partner in a person's plan for a fuller, healthier life.

BOTTOM LINE: "The doctor that resides within" each of us will take on a more important role sooner than later. Get to know that doctor. Someday he may save your life!

# PLACEBO

*Placebo* is Latin for "I shall please." Sometime back around the 14th century it meant "flatterer," "toady," or "bootlicker." In the late 18th century, when the word *placebo* entered medical terminology, the disdainful meaning stuck, and *placebo* was defined as a medicine given to please, rather than benefit, patients. Well, that isn't quite what we understand today.

A powerful part of healing, the placebo effect contributes to the success of many treatments. The placebo effect can be a great ally to doctors and patients when used responsibly and under the right circumstances. There is nothing morally wrong with being responsible for a placebo.

Conditioning often plays a major roll in the placebo effect. Patients who have experienced relief by taking a medication may unconsciously associate aspects of the medication—like recognizing a white or blue pill—with relief.

Galen, a prominent Greek physician, surgeon and philosopher in the 2nd century said, "He cures most successfully in whom the people have the most confidence." Confidence is the major power factor that produces the placebo effect. People feel confident and secure when they are in the hands of a respected, recognized mentor. Recognition is an indispensable ingredient in placebo treatment. External trappings such as diplomas, board certifications, even fancy signs add to the placebo effect.

Placebo power also comes from expectations. Often, when we choose the more expensive of two options, we have greater expectations, and sometimes, our expectations become reality simply because of the placebo effect. When a close friend or relative recommends a service from another person, that also carries with it greater expectations.

Should physicians prescribe drugs or procedures that they know to be of no intrinsic value in order to take advantage of the placebo effect? Good question. As an example, at least a portion of the benefit of antidepressants comes the placebo effect. But deliberate placebo therapy presents what has seemed to be an insolvable medical-ethical dilemma: If a physician tells a patient that a sugar pill has been prescribed, the placebo response, which depends in part on patients' expectations of receiving a plausible treatment, will be lost. But if physicians tell patients that a pharmacologically active medicine has been prescribed, they are engaging in deception that is neither ethical nor, in the long run, therapeutic.

Most physicians see placebos, like many conventional drugs, as broadly effective therapies whose mechanisms of action are not completely understood and which tend to be more useful for some conditions than others. In reality, measurable physiological changes do occur from the prescribed substance. A placebo often has a life of its own—that is, after a short period of time most placebos lose the major portion of their benefit, and then the "real time" efficacy, or lack of it, takes hold.

The ultimate placebo, in my own medical history, was my mother's mustard plaster. She mixed powdered mustard and flour in water to concoct the century-old formula, and then she put it between two fabrics (I think it was the flour sack itself) and applied it to my chest when I was sick. Burn, sure did, but her gentle hands and concerned countenance, along with the highly placebotized therapy, always brought me back to health. To this day, I am looking for that formula. I would have liked to try it on my patients.

BOTTOM LINE: Confidence in and expectations of the placebo are the major power that produces the placebo effect.

# THE COST OF DYING

In 2009, Steve Kroft interviewed Dr. Ira Byock and Dr. Elliott Fisher on an episode of *60 Minutes* called "The Cost of Dying," and this chapter was inspired by that interview.

The interview begins:
*Last year, Medicare paid $55 billion in doctor and hospital bills that covered the last two months of patients' lives. That's more than the budget for either the Department of Homeland Security or the Department of Education. And it has been estimated that 20 to 30 percent of these medical expenses may have had no meaningful impact. Most of the bills were paid for by the federal government.[121]*

Of patients in the U.S., Fisher says, "They're likely to be seen by a dozen or more specialists who will conduct all kinds of tests, whether they're essential or not. Selectively reducing treatments and procedures which have little influence on quality of life and longevity must be addressed with vigor and resolve. This would reduce governmental cost."[122] If you have ever visited an intensive care floor at the hospital, either as a patient or visitor, you have probably noticed crowds of jacketed persons huddled around a computer at the nurses station—specialists called in to ponder, then treat, then ponder again, then re-treat each ICU patient. I have heard critically ill patients speak of doctors they saw only once, never knowing why they were there or what subspecialty they represented. One patient may see as many as 10 to 15 doctors and consultants during an ICU stay.

Clearly a significant portion of the dollar spent on the aging population is for critical care, and that critical care is often given in the ICU setting or in skilled nursing facilities. The last month of life is particularly expensive for Medicare and the patient.

Helen Adamopoulos, in "The Cost and Quality Conundrum of American End-of-Life Care," published on the Medicare Newsgroup website:

*Medicare spends an average of $6,620 in the last month of a beneficiary's life versus $325 for survivors, while the dying beneficiary spends an average of $588 out of pocket in their last month of life compared to survivors who spend an average of $126 per month, according to CMS (Centers for Medicare and Medicaid)*

---

[121] http://www.cbsnews.com/news/the-cost-of-dying/

[122] http://www.cbsnews.com/news/the-cost-of-dying/

*data available from 1992-1999. On average, Medicare spends*
*$20,870 per beneficiary who dies while in the hospital.*[123]

This propensity to try to rescue the dying patient is not going to go away anytime soon, and indeed may be increasing in momentum.

The intensive care unit (ICU) is where the best of minds, the best of equipment, and the most advanced life-saving work occurs. It is also the most expensive hotel in town, costing around $10,000 per 24-hour stay. By law, Medicare cannot reject the payment of any treatment based upon cost. "Breakfast in bed" is most often intravenous infusion of dextrose (sugar) in water. More than 25 percent of Medicare spending goes toward the five percent of beneficiaries who die each year.[124] Unlike the standard short-stay facility (the Marriott, for example), care in the ICU may be rendered for many days or weeks, again with a tab near $10,000 per day.

"This is the way so many Americans die. Something like 18 to 20 percent of Americans spend their last days in an ICU," Byock told Kroft in the 60 Minutes interview, "And, you know, it's extremely expensive. It's uncomfortable. Many times they have to be sedated so that they don't reflexively pull out a tube, or sometimes their hands are restrained. This is not the way most people would want to spend their last days of life. And yet, this has become almost the medical last rites for people as they die." Kroft pointed out, "There are people that would argue that this is great medicine. You get tested for every conceivable, possible malady you might have."[125]

The U.S. medical system seems top-heavy in ICU units. The United States has 25 ICU beds per 100,000 people, while the United Kingdom has only 5 per 100,000—yet our outcomes are no better.

If you stick your head into an intensive care unit, you will be overwhelmed with all the monitors, tubes, cables, bells, whistles, and beepings. What do they all mean? I don't know. I am just hoping all the super specialists, various technicians, nurses, hospitalists, etc., *do* know.

What are the wishes of those who actually are the recipients of this system we administer? A vast majority of Americans say they want to die at home, but 75 percent die in a hospital or a nursing home.

How we treat end-of-life folks is deeply ingrained in our system.

Compare this to the hospice environment. Hospice gives medical, psychological, and spiritual support to the dying patient and family. In my own very limited personal experience, I'd say that a hospice provided a more comfortable atmosphere and left my wife, at the end of her life, better cared for at

---

[123] http://www.medicarenewsgroup.com/context/understanding-medicare-blog/understanding-medicare-blog/2013/06/03/the-cost-and-quality-conundrum-of-american-end-of-life-care

[124] http://www.medicarenewsgroup.com/context/understanding-medicare-blog/understanding-medicare-blog/2013/06/03/the-cost-and-quality-conundrum-of-american-end-of-life-care

[125] http://www.cbsnews.com/news/the-cost-of-dying/

home than she would have been in an ICU unit.

Hospice is but a part of the U.S. health care system's end-of-life care puzzle. Hospice is far from perfect, and at times may not seem to fit as well as one might want it to fit in the scheme of health care. However, my experience as a physician working closely with hospice was good, and I was both grateful and impressed by the compassion and skill shown by the team of healthcare professionals and volunteers. The goal of the care is to help people who are dying have peace, comfort, and dignity.

BOTTOM LINE: The present-day approach to caring for the end-of-life patient has evolved into a complex conundrum whose solution is equally as daunting. We have both the will and means for doing what is right and morally correct. We just need to be about it sooner rather than later.

# TOOLS

From Steve Maraboli's book *Life, the Truth, and Being Free*: "Accept yourself, your strengths, your weaknesses, your truths, and know what tools you have to fulfill your purpose."[126]

My intent is not to write a great philosophical treatise on tools, but only mention that in this book are tools you can gather and use as part of your armamentarium. To sharpen the tools, re-read sections that you find useful. When a tool has served its purpose, you may elect to discard it.

One of the greatest quests I have in my life is for tools—the right tools for the right jobs. To be more effective, I need to know what tools are available and whether they are fitted for the specific job, which is ahead of me. Sometimes I find out the answer only when I use the tool.

Some years ago, in the middle of my medical career, my wife and I and another couple were driving down to the Boulder Mountain area in Utah to do some fishing. We had an old Ford station wagon, which was about ready for a trade-in. Halfway to our destination, I stopped to check out a rattle, and while we were parked at the side of the road I saw a wire fence bordering a pasture. There was an unattached piece of bailing wire on one of the fence posts. Not having a good reason, I confiscated the wire and put it in the trunk. The trip continued.

As we got closer to the fishing area, it became darker and the road became bumpier. I understood speed and what it could do for us in getting us to the right place at the right time. In this case, the right time would be before it got too dark.

It wasn't long until I developed considerable skills in avoiding rocks, ruts, and chuckholes. The old Ford station wagon began to look and feel more like a tank. Unfortunately, believing that became my mentality.

Deep in the forest, it was getting dark. I crested a hill, came down into a small dip in the road, and without so much as a warning crunch or screech of metal, we suddenly lost the gas tank as I "high-centered" the vehicle. To my amazement, I found out the Ford was not a tank!

I'm sure most everyone understands that cars don't run very far without gas tanks attached, no matter how full the gas tank is. We pushed the car off to the side of the road and bedded down for the evening. Morning came, and the least of our worries was whether the fish were biting or not.

After my third set of apologies, and my wife's fourth set of "I told you so's," my friend and I—mostly my friend—began to put the gas tank on the car. Our search for the appropriate tools, of course, yielded only bailing wire. We had lost the gas cap, so my hanky served to take its place. With some faith (the

---

[126] *The Power of One*, Steve Maraboli, A Better Today Publishing (December 1, 2010)

women provided that), prayers (mostly by me), and the bailing wire, we made it out of the mountains.

Ever since then, I have understood the appropriateness of tools and their usage. I have seen some of my friends who make a habit of collecting tools. They have so many tools in their garage and shop that I can't imagine where they all came from. And don't you know, these are the people who never have anything break down. You may believe that your present life is "broken down," yet have hope that the tools and new resolve to make your future what it should be will put you back on he road to "good fishing" (optimal health).

"Today, you have the opportunity to transcend from a disempowered mindset of existence to an empowered reality of purpose-driven living. Today is a new day that has been handed to you for shaping. You have the tools, now get out there and create a masterpiece." — Steve Maraboli[127]

BOTTOM LINE: You will have the tools to shape your health future, "Now get out there and create a masterpiece."

[127] *The Power of One*, Steve Maraboli, A Better Today Publishing (December 1, 2010)

# NONCOMPLIANCE

The assumption that physicians know what they are doing is a pretty safe one, in general. If you are not sure that is the case in your relationship with your physician, ask questions or seek a different caregiver. Once your faith in your physician is secure, then it is wise to follow his or her instructions.

In following instructions, we use the word *compliance*. Compliance implies that patients follow instructions given to them by their caregivers in managing their medical conditions. *Noncompliance*, as you have properly assumed, is not following instructions. Noncompliance is one of the most pressing problems we are faced with in our attempts to deliver optimal care to patients. Noncompliance, or poor compliance, is estimated to cost the U.S. healthcare system $290 billion a year.[128] Poor medication compliance is implicated in over 125,000 U.S. deaths per year.[129] A compliance discussion fits into any healthy lifestyle program.

As you proceed with the suggestions and information I will give you and undertake whatever lifestyle changes are necessary, you have to be your own doctor in the sense that you must periodically review your degree of compliance. Chart your own course.

To be labeled as noncompliant does not in itself tell us why instructions were not followed. There are a lot of chances for miscommunication. There were about 3.8 billion prescriptions written in the year 2013. Over 50 percent of prescriptions were taken incorrectly or not at all.[130]

As concerning prescriptions, noncompliance could include one or a combination of any of the following:

1. Failing to fill a new or old prescription—not thinking the medication is important or believing the prescription to be too expensive
2. Failing to follow instructions on how to take medication
3. Carelessness in routine, quantity, and frequency of use of medication
4. Inability, for whatever reason, to follow the instructions—arthritis of hands, tremors, or mental confusion
5. Losing or misplacing the prescription or the medication
6. Previous adverse reaction to the same or other medications

As former Surgeon General C. Everett Koop put it so succinctly, "Drugs don't work in people who don't take them."[131] It is surprising how pervasive noncompliance is. The following statistics were printed in *American Medical News:*

---

[128] http://www.nehi.net/bendthecurve/sup/documents/Medication_Adherence_Brief.pdf

[129] http://www.medscape.com/viewarticle/818850

[130] http://www.medscape.com/viewarticle/818850

[131] http://www.nejm.org/doi/full/10.1056/NEJMra050100

1. 75 percent of patients sometimes fail to take their medications as directed.
2. 33 percent of prescriptions are never filled.
3. 50 percent to 60 percent of the time, patients with chronic conditions do not take their medications.
4. 33 percent to 69 percent of medication-related hospitalizations are linked to drug non-adherence.
5. 125,000 patient deaths each year are linked to drug noncompliance.
6. $290 billion is spent annually on care needed because of medication noncompliance.[132]

Not too infrequently, the physician is at fault when patients don't take their medications correctly. In the article "Why Are So Many Patients Noncompliant," *Medscape Family Medicine* printed the results of a survey that showed that in 10 to 39 percent of prescriptions, physicians fail to give medication instructions. They discuss dosing directions in fewer than 60 percent of new prescriptions cases. And they review potential adverse events only 33 percent of the time. "But the larger problem is that too little information is offered to patients who want and need more. The average time that a doctor spends discussing all aspects of a newly prescribed medication is a mere 49 seconds."[133]

As you commit to and undertake any of the programs, suggestions, or protocols in this book, as with any other treatment, you need to be compliant in order for them to work. Please view your behavioral changes in that light.

BOTTOM LINE: Check with your doctor before changing or stopping any of your medication. Be adherent and compliant in your lifestyle plans to improve your health status.

---

[132] http://www.medscape.com/viewarticle/818850
[133] http://www.medscape.com/viewarticle/818850_4

# ORGANIC FOODS

An organic food, by definition, is a food produced with no synthetic inputs such as pesticides, fertilizers, or antibiotics. Organic food sales have dramatically increased and are projected to reach 28.4 billion dollars in sales in 2014.[134]

Organic foods are expensive, and that is a definite disadvantage. But are they worth the extra cost? Let's see if we can find out.

There have been 237 well-designed, well-analyzed studies on organic versus conventional foods. Off the bat, there are a couple of problems with trying to study the difference in the two categories. The first, among the 237 studies, was a high variability in the ways and methods used to draw firm conclusions. Additionally, there are no long-term follow up studies to tell us what to expect down the road from ingesting organic foods. That is always important in the study of anything that we ingest—food, dietary supplements, or medications

In the 237 studies on organic food, in general, the nutritional benefits from vitamins and minerals was essentially the same in the organic versus the conventional group, except that phosphorus was found in greater amounts in organic foods, and omega-3 was more prevalent in organic milk and chicken. Regarding the contamination of mercury and arsenic, no significant difference was found between conventional food and organic foods. Pesticide residue was studied, and was found to be 7 percent in organic vs. 37 percent in conventional food. However, conventional food with pesticide residue was still within government guidelines. With pathogenic bacteria (the "bad guys"), there was no difference. When bacterial resistance was found, it was 33 percent higher in conventional chicken and pork than it was in organic chicken and pork.[135]

BOTTOM LINE: Eating organic food, that is up to you. Will you live a better and longer life? I don't know. At this point, I don't think anyone does.

---

[134] http://www.ers.usda.gov/topics/natural-resources-environment/organic-agriculture/organic-market-overview.aspx#.U9_2elbfUQc

[135] http://med.stanford.edu/news/all-news/2012/09/little-evidence-of-health-benefits-from-organic-foods-study-finds.html

# SERVINGS AND PORTIONS

When shopping or doing food calculations, make sure to read the serving size for each food item, because there is often more than one serving in a package, and the nutritional content listed for any food is based on serving size. While the terms *serving* and *portion* often are used interchangeably, they actually mean different things. If portions fit the standards of measurement and are actual specific measurements, the information can be used in the same way as serving size information. A *serving* is the amount of food recommended in consumer education materials—a measured amount. A *portion* is the amount of a food you choose to eat at any one meal or snack

An example of a measured serving is one slice of bread or one 8-ounce cup of milk. Many dietary programs and food lists talk of portions, such as the list you will see below. I think people care about what is in the products they buy, but they may not understand the information—or more likely, they don't take the time to read labels. I once read a Mayo Clinic report that an average shopper in a grocery store looks at 61 items in 26 minutes. That doesn't leave much time to scrutinize labels. But reading labels could literally be a lifesaver.

A package size is a single food container. Package size contents can be misleading. Many foods, particularly beverage items, come in a single container containing two or more servings. A bottle of soda might list its nutritional content as containing just 80 calories per serving, but if a serving size is 20 ounces, that soda actually contains 200 calories, not 80.

As a rough guide, one portion (and in this case is also a serving size) is measured as:

- 3 heaping tablespoons of cooked vegetables like broccoli or carrots
- A small bowl of salad vegetables like lettuce or spinach
- A medium-sized piece of fruit like an apple or a banana
- A slice of large fruit like melon
- A handful of smaller fruit like grapes
- A tablespoon of dried fruit like raisins
- 2 pieces of small fruit like plums
- 3 heaping tablespoons of food such as chickpeas or baked beans
- A small glass (150ml) of pure fruit juice
- A 3-ounce piece of cooked meat, about the size of a deck of cards—for instance, half a chicken breast or a chicken leg without the thigh or skin
- ¾ cup of flaked fish
- 2 thin slices of lean roast beef

The American Heart Association lists the following serving-size information:[136]

**Grains:**
- 1 slice of bread
- 1 ounce of ready-to-eat cereal
- ½ cup of cooked cereal, rice, or pasta (about the size of half a baseball)
- A half a bagel

**Vegetables:**
- 1 cup of raw leafy vegetables (about the size of a small fist)
- 1/2 cup of other vegetables
- 1/2 cup of vegetable juice

**Fruits:**
- 1 medium fruit (medium is defined as the size of a baseball)
- ½ cup chopped, cooked, or canned fruit
- ½ cup juice

**Meat, Poultry, Fish, Dry Beans, and Nuts:**
- 2 to 3 ounces of cooked lean meat, poultry, or fish
- ½ cup cooked dry beans
- 2 tablespoons of peanut butter
- 3 ounces of cooked lean meat or poultry (about the size of a computer mouse)

**Milk, Yogurt, and Cheese:**
- 1 cup of fat-free or low-fat milk or yogurt
- 1 ½ ounces fat-free or low-fat cheese

Here are some everyday comparisons to help you figure out serving sizes:

- An ounce and a half of cheese is the size of four stacked dice.
- 3 ounces of meat is the size of a deck of cards.
- ½ cup of fresh fruit is the size of a tennis ball.
- A cup of pasta is the size of a baseball.
- A thumb equals 1 teaspoon.
- One small fist (cupped hand) is a serving size, or is equivalent to 1 cup.
- One hockey puck is a serving.

If a diet or set of instructions tells you to eat "seven to ten servings daily" of a type of food, say fruits and vegetables, you may choose among many types,

---

136 http://www.heart.org/HEARTORG/GettingHealthy/NutritionCenter/HealthyEating/Suggested-Servings-from-Each-Food-Group_UCM_318186_Article.jsp

always keeping variety in mind: apricots, broccoli, chard, carrots, mangoes, oranges, peaches, tomatoes, corn, spinach, grapefruit, apples, red grapes. But if you have a special liking for one food, like broccoli, you can always "double up." Or even triple.

Average portion sizes have grown considerably over the past 20 years. You can take a restaurant entrée and split it with someone and still come away well fed. This mindset has been aptly labeled "portion distortion."

Check out these examples of how larger portions lead to increased calories:

**Chart furnished by the National Institute of Health**
**Comparison of Portions and Calories 20 Years Ago to Present Day[137]**

|  | 20 Years Ago | | Today | |
|---|---|---|---|---|
|  | Portion | Calories | Portion | Calorie |
| Bagel | 3" diameter | 140 | 6" diameter | 350 |
| Cheeseburger | 1 | 333 | 1 | 590 |
| Spaghetti w/meatballs | 1 cup sauce 3 small meatballs | 500 | 2 cups sauce 3 large meatballs | 1,020 |
| Soda | 6.5 ounces | 82 | 20 ounces | 250 |
| Blueberry muffin | 1.5 ounces | 210 | 5 ounces | 500 |

---

[137] http://www.nhlbi.nih.gov/health/educational/wecan/eat-right/distortion.htm

# FAST FOODS AND THE INFLUENCE OF TV

Could the solution to our dietary problems be to shut down all fast food establishments? Might be a good idea, but unlikely any time soon to be on any legislative agenda. If you look at the list of the top five sources of caloric intake in the USA, you can see why I asked the question. These food items account for about a fifth of all calories consumed in the U.S.

1. Sugared beverages (7 percent of total): a 20-oz. soda contains 66 grams of sugar, or about 17 tsp. (250 kcals). (Just think of kcals as calories.)
2. Cake and sweet rolls
3. Hamburgers and cheeseburgers
4. Pizza
5. Potato and corn chips

You may be thinking that the fast-food "eat and run" restaurant is a modern day revelation, but records indicate that the fast-food shop was actually created in large ancient cities. The urban Roman ate from street stalls that served various meats and breads, and the wines offered to the customer were usually thinned with water. The oldest known fast-food shop was found in the Sumerian city of Ur. It was in business in 1800 B.C. I wonder if they had our ever so prevalent "drive-through," but with horses or chariots?

Over the last few years, the "super-sizing" phenomenon and highly processed foods (which includes extra portions of salt) have penetrated all of our lives, to the detriment of good health.

What fast foods are: calorie dense, plagued with saturated fats, often containing trans fats, high in sugar—and obviously "fast," which fits well into our on-the-go culture. Fast foods are also relatively inexpensive in terms of calories delivered per dollar spent.

Let's first attack the beverage conundrum. American adults put into their stomachs 15 percent of their calories from sugars added during the processing of foods. Sugar-sweetened beverages account for 37 percent of that total intake. Studies tells us that regularly drinking as little as one 12-ounce sugary soda a day could increase the risk of cardiovascular disease by about 30 percent, independent of total calories, obesity, or other risk factors.[138]

Take a look at some of our common beverages. Take a long look.

| | | |
|---|---|---|
| Coke | 12-oz | 140 calories |
| Coke | 20-oz | 240 calories |
| 7-Eleven Big Gulp | 32-oz | 364 calories |

---

[138] http://www.medscape.com/viewarticle/820172

| 7-Eleven Double Gulp | 44-oz | 744 calories |
| Mountain Dew | 20-oz | 290 calories |
| Orange Juice | 16-oz | 220 calories[139] |

Would it surprise you to know that the adolescent obesity problem in our country is not due to excess pizza or hamburgers—though they do contribute—but to sugary beverages? If a teenager were to consume one 20-ounce bottle of soda a day (not an unusual scenario), she would consume 87,660 calories in one year. That translates into an additional whopping 25 pounds! Twenty-five pounds of pure empty calories distributed on hips, buttock, belly, and abdominal organs. That is simply disastrous, and the adverse effects may appear sooner than later. Sooner: insulin intolerance/diabetes. Later: cardiovascular disease.

Next, the burger: A super-sized burger meal can have as many as 2,300 calories, about the number of calories burned when running a marathon. This is an example of not only a high calorie food, but also one that is injurious to our body because of its fat content. Keep in mind that it is the saturated fat that is most harmful to the vessels of our body.

**Nutritional facts about a Big Mac:**
| Total calories | 550 calories |
| Calories from fat | 260 calories[140] |
| Carbohydrates | 47 grams[141] |

Fast food breakfasts can also be disastrous in terms of calories and ingredients. I have selected a few meals just to give you an example and feeling for the calorie and salt content. Remember, excess salt intake may lead to cardiovascular disease.

This chart was borrowed from the website http://fast-food-nutrition.findthebest.com/d/a/Breakfast. There is a lot of great information on this site about what goes past your teeth and reaches your bloodstream.[142]

| Fast Food Restaurant | Calories | Salt, in mg |
| --- | --- | --- |
| Hardee's Monster Biscuit | 1,720 | 2,180 |
| McDonald's Big Breakfast with Hotcakes (Large Size Biscuit) | 1,150 | |
| McDonald's Sausage McMuffin with Egg | 450 | 2,260 |
| Burger King BK Ultimate | 1,450 | 2,920 |

---

[139] http://www.sugarstacks.com/beverages.htm

[140] http://fast-food-nutrition.findthebest.com/l/8/McDonald-s-Big-Mac

[141] http://nutritiondata.self.com/facts/foods-from-mcdonalds/6220/2

[142] http://fast-food-nutrition.findthebest.com

| Breakfast Platter | | |
| --- | --- | --- |
| Sonic Ultimate Meat & Cheese Breakfast Burrito | 800 | 2,140 |
| Subway FOOTLONG™ Bread Steak & Cheese | 860 | 2,380 |

At fast food restaurants, almost everything that goes into that basket or thin paper-wrap is freeze-dried, frozen, canned, or dehydrated. Your food has been super-sized with super amounts of saturated fats and highly processed carbohydrates, not to mention more animal protein than is good for you. Your meal has been cooked at very high temperatures, further potentiating the bad effects, with lard or vegetable oils.

People analyze their food purchase on the basis of four considerations:
1. Taste
2. Cost
3. Convenience
4. Health

Health, unfortunately, is the least of a buyer's concerns. Why should we be concerned about the health properties of a food that looks so good, smells so good, and better yet, tastes so good?

In a study of 5,731 adult and older men and women, a research team at Psychosomatic Medicine found a lower risk of depression among participants with better-quality diets, and increased anxiety was observed with a higher intake of processed and unhealthy foods.[143]

**The Often Subtle Influence of Television**

Television advertising is a big industry and has a wide influence on its watchers. A research article in JAMA (*The Journal of the American Medical Association*) reports that every hour increase in television viewing is associated with consumption of an additional 167 calorie each day.[144] Seems like a lot, but that is what they reported. This increase in energy consumption was accounted for by the foods commonly advertised on television, including salty and sweet snacks and fast food. In eating what they watch, children eat more plentiful amounts and less healthy food.

I will give you information on how television influences our children, but adults also sit—or lay—themselves in front of the TV and are subject to the same covert and overt messages viewed on the set. Yale University's Rudd Center for Food Policy and Obesity reported that children and adults alike who watch ads for food on TV, especially ones for unhealthy products, are more likely to snack

---

[143] http://www.medscape.com/viewarticle/819974

[144] http://jama.jamanetwork.com/article.aspx?articleid=202652

on those foods, and are potentially at a higher risk for obesity.[145] I don't find that information to be too revealing, as I assumed as much, many years ago.

Research has documented the massive amounts of television that our children view. The University of Michigan Health System gives us the following figures:

- On average, children ages two to five spend 32 hours a week in front of a TV set watching television, DVDs, DVR, and videos or using a game console.
- Kids ages six to eleven spend about 28 hours a week in front of the TV.
- 71 percent of eight to eighteen-year-olds have a TV in their bedroom.
- In about two-thirds of households, the TV is usually on during meals.
- In 53 percent of households with seventh to twelfth graders, there are no rules about TV watching.
- The average child sees more than 40,000 commercials a year.[146]

Along with all the noise, clatter, and sometimes edifying programs comes a supersized main course of commercials. The amount of commercials in prime-time programming has steadily increased so that today 36 percent of our viewing is of commercials. The combined load of brand appearances and network ad messages in late night shows is thirty seconds shy of a half-hour, or 49 percent of total content time. During Saturday morning cartoons, children view an average of one food commercial every five minutes. More than 90 percent of these advertisements are for high-sugar cereals and candy bars, salty canned foods, fast food, or other junk food.[147]

The American Academy of Pediatrics (AAP) recommends that children under age two not watch any television, and that older kids not spend more than two hours a day watching TV or otherwise using a screen (via DVDs, video games, computer use not related to school, tablets, and smart phones). Also, the content of what they do view should be nonviolent and educational.

As part of your program, I want you to consider stopping any future visits to fast-food restaurants until you gain control and develop wisdom. Unanticipated straying from your dead-on determination to stay away from fast foods is dangerous. "Just this once" is poison to any program that you are trying to follow.

BOTTOM LINE: Fast food is a modern convenience you can do without. TV is a double-edged sword. Make rules, limit TV, and stick to your rules.

---

[145] http://www.marketingcharts.com/television/tv-junk-food-ads-trigger-automatic-eating-9709/

[146] http://www.med.umich.edu/yourchild/topics/tv.htm

[147] http://www.med.umich.edu/yourchild/topics/tv.htm

# SUGARS

Centuries ago, sugar was produced only from sugarcane, so it was rather expensive and not extensively used. In 1812, sugar began to be extracted from beets, and the prices came down.

At the beginning of the 19th century, the French consumed approximately 1.6 pounds per person each year. As its popularity and availability increased, more and more sugar was eaten. French consumption in 1880 was 16 pounds a year per person. It rose to 34 pounds per person in 1900, and 80 pounds per person in 1960. Even so, at that point, the French still consumed less sugar than the rest of the Western world.

In terms of energy furnished per cost, sugar is near the top of the list. But quite apart from its value as a food, sugar has become important as a flavor in our diet. In fact, it's beloved much more for its agreeable flavor than for its physiological nutrient value. This favors overindulgence.

Sugar is the generalized name for sweet, soluble carbohydrates we consume. There are various types of sugar. Simple sugars are called monosaccharides and include glucose, fructose, and galactose. The table sugar most customarily used is sucrose, a disaccharide. The chart below breaks down the components found within particular sugars, as well as the caloric concentration and food source of these sugars.

| SUGAR | INGREDIENTS | CALORIES | FOUND IN |
|---|---|---|---|
| sucrose | glucose/fructose | 16 cal/tsp. | fruits, veg, honey, corn syrup, powdered sugar |
| honey | glucose/fructose | 22 cal/tsp. | honey |
| glucose | Glucose | 16 cal/tsp. | corn syrup, maple syrup |
| maltose (malt sugar) | from fermented starch (corn) | 16 cal/tsp. | cereal, baked goods, beer |
| sugar alcohols | sorbitol, mannitol, xylitol, maltitol (from fruits or commercial dextrose) | 9-12 cal/tsp. | chocolate, candies, chewing gum, jam, some table syrups |
| lactose (milk) sugar | glucose/lactose | 16/cal/tsp. | milk |

When a product claims to be "sugar free," that usually means it does not contain sucrose. "Sugar free" doesn't mean no calories or low calories, so keep your eye on that one.

Let's look a little deeper into the sugar bowl. A study reported in the *Journal of the American Medical Association* in February 2014 called "Added Sugar Intake and Cardiovascular Diseases Mortality Among U.S. Adults" reported research conducted under the direction of Quanhe Yang about U.S. consumption of added sugar. Probably not to anyone's surprise, our consumption of added sugar is excessive. In persons two years or older, the 1977 caloric intake was 235 calories a day, while from 1994 to 1996, the figure was 318 calories a day. Based on a 2,000-calorie diet, in 2010 the average American consumed about 15 percent of daily calories from added sugar.[148]

That's considerably in excess of what the American Heart Association recommends. Their recommendation is that women consume no more than 100 calories a day from added sugars, and men consume no more than 150 calories.[149]

For the purposes of the sugar study cited above, "added sugars" include all sugars added in the processing or preparing of foods. This includes sugar-sweetened beverages, fruit drinks, grain-based desserts, dairy desserts, candy, ready-to-eat cereals, and yeast breads. Understandably, naturally occurring sugars, such as in fruits and fruit juices, were not included in the study.

Throughout this book, I've noted many pitfalls of sugar consumption, including its role in causing and exacerbating weight problems. In addition, excess carbohydrates, particularly the fructose in soda beverages, increase triglycerides and can cause injury to the liver. Excessive sugar intake is the roadway to diabetes and obesity, with its myriad of pathological states. And there is a significant relationship between added sugar consumption and increased risk for CVD (cardiovascular disease) mortality.

Luckily, there are many situations where artificial sweeteners can be substituted in place of sugar. Artificial sweeteners include saccharin, aspartame, cyclamate, sucralose, acesulfame potassium, and stevia. Current knowledge reports these are safe, and I find them important in my own dietary program. Taste-wise, I have a difficult time differentiating artificial sweeteners from the "real stuff."

BOTTOM LINE: Good judgment calls for avoiding all added sugars.

---

[148] http://archinte.jamanetwork.com/issue.aspx?journalid=71&issueid=929736

[149] http://www.heart.org/HEARTORG/GettingHealthy/NutritionCenter/HealthyDietGoals/Frequently-Asked-Questions-About-Sugar_UCM_306725_Article.jsp

# FRUIT JUICES

For the average person, examining daily caloric intake yields a substantial portion of calories coming from non-alcoholic beverages like carbonated drinks, soda, and juices. A six- to eight-ounce glass of orange juice each morning, though traditional, may not be the best way to start the morning. I will try to show you why.

Real fruit juice has a similar sugar content as sugar-sweetened beverages; as an example, eight and a half ounces of apple juice contains 26 grams of sugar and a total of 110 calories. The same amount of a cola drink contains 105 kcals and 26 ½ grams of sugar—essentially the same.

A February 2014 study reported in *The Lancet Diabetes & Endocrinology* showed that consumption of 16 ounces of high-antioxidant Concord grape juice a day for three months increased insulin resistance and waist circumference in overweight adults. (Insulin resistance is the metabolic precursor to diabetes.) We know that waist circumference is a manifestation of increased intra-abdominal fat, a condition with a higher correlation to earlier morbidity and mortality.

Fruit juices and smoothies are not an alternative to sweetened beverages. Naveed Sattar, MD, professor of metabolic medicine at the Institute of Cardiovascular and Medical Sciences at the University of Glasgow, tells us that research is starting to show that high fruit juice consumption is closely tied to an increased risk for diabetes.[150]

BOTTOM LINE: Limit fruit juices, as well as soda pop, and satisfy that fruit taste preference with an apple instead.

---

[150] http://www.bmj.com/rapid-responses?sort_by=field_highwire_a_epubdate_value_1&sort_order=ASC&items_per_page=180&page=52 0

# FISH

Eating fish will help lower your risk of heart disease. The current recommendation from The U.S. Food and Drug Administration (FDA) and the U.S. Environmental Protection Agency (EPA) is that we eat at least two servings of fish each week. To maximize the beneficial effects of eating fish, you should make your selections from this list of oily fish: salmon, mackerel, herring, sardines, tuna, and lake trout. Avoid fish with mercury: swordfish, king mackerel, shark, or tilefish. I have never tasted any of these four, and at this point, I have no temptation to do so.

The desired nutrients in the fish are Eicosapentaenoic acid (EPA) and Docosahexaenoic acid (DHA). EPA is an omega-3 fatty acid and a polyunsaturated fatty acid (PUFA). DHA is an omega-3 fatty acid and is the most abundant fatty acid in our brains. As a matter of fact, there is a whole lot of it in there. Cold-water oceanic fish oils are rich in DHA. Poultry and eggs provide lower amount of EPA and DHA.

Alpha-linolenic acid , or ALA, has similar benefits and is derived from plants. Not to be confused with linoleic acid, ALA is an essential omega-3 fatty acid and organic compound found in seeds such as nuts (notably walnuts) and many common vegetable oils, such as soybean and canola oil. The body can convert ALA into DHA.

These three nutrients, when derived from their natural sources, have unquestionable positive benefits on human health. It is important that you have picked up on "natural source," as supplemental omega-3 fatty acids may incur no benefit to vessels.

Listed below are some popular fish types and their approximate total content of fatty acids, in four-ounce portions. You will want to choose the fish with the highest amount of fatty acid. However, availability, cost, and taste preference may override that decision:

Anchovies: 2,300-2,400 mg
Cod: 200 mg
Salmon (Atlantic, Chinook, Coho): 1,200-2,400 mg
Sardines: 1,100-1,600 mg
Scallops: 200 mg
Trout: 1,000-1,100 mg
Tilapia: 150 mg
Yellow fin *tuna: 150-350, canned: 150-300 mg[151]

---

[151] http://health.usnews.com/health-news/diet-fitness/diet/articles/2011/04/14/8-easy-ways-to-load-up-on-healthy-omega-3-fats

Note that canned tuna comes from several varieties of tuna including Yellowfin and Bluefin (Hawaiians call it Ahi), which are labeled as "light meat," and Albacore, the only tuna that can be labeled "premium white meat." To get the most omega-3 fats from your canned tuna, choose water-packed tuna rather than oil-packed. Canned in water and drained, six ounces of light-meat tuna typically provides a little less than 500 mg. of omega-3 fatty acids, while light tuna canned in oil and drained provides a little more than 300 mg. of omega- 3s.

Greenland Eskimos who consumed a diet high in omega-3 fatty acids had a lower incidence of coronary heart disease, heart attacks, and decreased tendencies for abnormal blood clotting. Their diet is mostly seal and whale, which are high in fatty acids. Other cultures have shown similar results—that is, decreased cardiovascular disease with high omega-3 to omega-6 fatty acid ratios.[152]

Many studies report that omega-3 fatty acids may help reduce blood pressure, but the benefits have generally been small. Also, fish oil has been reported to lessen the propensity for wrinkles on your skin. That's always a plus. Right ladies? There have been studies conducted over a short period of time reporting improvements in rheumatoid arthritis and the benefits of decreased morning stiffness and joint tenderness. Fish oil probably works on the immune system in people with rheumatoid arthritis.

Now, we will dig deeper into the cholesterol arena. There is strong scientific evidence that omega-3 fatty acids from fish, or when indicated, fish oil supplements, can significantly reduce triglyceride levels. Higher doses have been found to have greater effects. Four grams daily may lower triglyceride levels up to 40 percent. This is one of the exceptions to the idea that I have addressed that supplements are not beneficial in preventing and treating cardiovascular disease. The benefit comes through lowering triglycerides and inflammation. Daily intake has been linked to a reduced risk of sudden heart failure. Often, when people have high triglycerides, they may also receive a prescription of a highly concentrated omega-3 fatty acids medicine taken from fish.

The most common complaint about taking fish oil supplements is the fishy burps or aftertaste. You can often avoid this side effect by taking the capsule frozen. This slows the breakdown of fish oil in your stomach, often reducing fishy burps. Take the capsule at the start of the meal. The food traps the fish oil in the stomach, and they mix together, buffering the odor. You might try switching brands as another way of overcoming these side effects. Pure omega-fatty acids don't have a fishy taste.

---

[152] http://www.mercola.com/beef/omega3_oil.htm

# VEGETABLES

Vegetables, along with fruits and whole grains, are the healthiest foods you can eat. The positive health benefits of a diet rich in vegetables and fruits have been proven over and over. The list of diseases altered by vegetables includes heart disease, stroke, some forms of cancers, eye disease, and digestive problems, and vegetables also smooth out the absorption of carbohydrates into the bloodstream. That is particularly good for those with insulin resistance and blood sugar abnormalities, such as obesity, pre-diabetes, and diabetes. An additional advantage: vegetables produce a greater feeling of fullness, and the time-to-hunger after eating is blunted by their intake.

**A Closer Look at Cancer and the Positive Effect Vegetables Have upon Cancer**

Two hundred studies examined the relationship between fruit and vegetable intake and cancers of the lung, colon, breast, cervix, esophagus, oral cavity, stomach, bladder, pancreas, and ovary. For most cancer sites, persons with low fruit and vegetable intake (at least the lower one-fourth of the population) experience about twice the risk of cancer compared with those with high intake. That should be a strong motivating factor to increase your consumption of fruits and vegetables.[153]

Another report tells us that , according to a global meta-analysis of 20 studies published over the last 19 years, eating 200 grams of fruits and vegetables each day may reduce stroke risk. After reviewing data of 760,629 individuals who had a combined 16,981 strokes, researchers noted a 32 percent reduction in stroke risk with 200 grams of daily fruit consumption and an 11 percent decrease with every 200 grams of daily vegetable intake.[154]

Fruits, in particular, were significantly protective in cancers of the esophagus, oral cavity, and larynx. There was strong evidence that cancer of the pancreas, stomach, colon, bladder, cervix, ovary, uterus, and breast were decreased by consumption of fruits and vegetables. In short, it's safe to say that substantially increasing consumption of these foods would lead to major public health benefits.

Increasing fruit and vegetable intake may be particularly beneficial in older people in terms of preventing stroke. All ages should strive to eat at least five to eight portions of a variety of fruits and vegetables per day. Additional benefit could be obtained with an intake of ten portions. My feeling about this is that ten is the figure we should aim for.

---

[153] PMID: 1408943 [PubMed - indexed for MEDLINE] http://www.ncbi.nlm.nih.gov/pubmed/1408943
[154] http://www.sciencedaily.com/releases/2014/05/140508172221.htm

In a European study, 313,074 men and women were followed for eight years. Those who ate at least eight servings of fruits and vegetables per day had a 22 percent lower risk of dying from coronary heart disease than those who ate fewer than three servings a day.[155]

Just a comment on fiber. As you have already learned, you will get good mileage out of adequate fiber intake. Try to get your fiber through vegetable and fruit consumption. Diets rich in foods containing fiber, such as some vegetables and fruits, reduce the risk of heart disease, obesity, and type 2 diabetes.

Eating vegetables and fruits rich in potassium as part of an overall healthy diet tends to lower blood pressure, and may also reduce the risk of developing kidney stones and help to decrease bone loss.

You need to eat vegetables every day, because you simply cannot find another food group that is as perfectly matched to our everyday human needs as vegetables.

The good news is that vegetables are so low in calories that it is very difficult to gain weight even if you overeat them. On average, you are looking at 50 calories (or less) per cup from most vegetables. That amount is astonishingly low. You need to eat vegetables every day, because they supply the necessary vitamins required by our bodies.

Finally, the pleasure of chewing and the amazing digestive benefits that come from a high-fiber diet should not be overlooked. Most people should aim for at least eight to ten servings (at least four cups) of vegetables and fruits a day, and potatoes don't count. Go for a variety of kinds and colors of produce to give your body the mix of nutrients it needs. Foods with color are superior because they have the greatest amounts of antioxidants.

---

[155] http://www.heartandstroke.com/site/pp.aspx?c=ikIQLcMWJtE&b=8782773&printmode=1

# FATS

We are striving to keep down our consumption of saturated fats and increase monounsaturated fats in our diets. As you can see, canola oil ranks high in being good fat; olive oil is a close second.

Research by Quynh Biu of UCSF shows us that reducing the intake of total or saturated fats decreases the risk of cardiovascular events by 22 percent in those patients who are able to sustain the modified diet for at least two years. Replacing saturated fats with monounsaturated and polyunsaturated fats reduces the risk of cardiovascular events, where replacing saturated fats with protein or carbohydrates (i.e., a low-fat diet) does not. Adherence to a reduced or modified-fat diet for at least six months resulted in a significant 14 percent decrease in the number of cardiovascular events. This risk reduction increased to 22 percent in those who followed the diet for two years or more.[156]

In practice, the most effective intervention should include not only advice and support for implementing a modified and reduced-fat diet, but also supplementation with more healthful, unsaturated fats.

You may remember the great 1970s discovery of fat's connection with coronary heart disease (CAD) . It was then reasonable to suggest that dietary treatment of CAD and weight-loss programs be based on a low-fat diet. So impressive were the studies that the American Heart Association and the American Diabetes Association became the cheerleaders of this movement.

We just didn't pay much attention to carbohydrates. In the 1970s, reducing fat seemed appropriate, and carbohydrate reduction took a very subordinate role. Fats are denser and include the bad saturated fats, which do the nasty things listed above.

Now, the current view is blame carbohydrates and fashion diets on a low-carbohydrate approach versus low fat. Indeed, low-fat diets are often more difficult to stick to. When it comes to weight loss, you will probably relate better to carbohydrates than fats. Once you have attained your goal, the long-term effort to keep pounds off should be to keep the fat intake down. The selection of a low-carbohydrate diet, when trying to lose weight, will result in a better cholesterol profile, and that can't be anything but good. A reminder: the focus on the low-carbohydrate diet should be on cutting down on dietary extrinsic sugars (sucrose and fructose) and starches.

**Fat Comparison Chart**

---

[156] Dietary Fat Modification And The Risk Of Future Cardiovascular Events And Mortality, Quynh Bui, UCSF
http://www.ncbi.nlm.nih.gov/pubmed/23668523

| Fat (1 Tbsp) gm. | Saturated | Monounsaturated | Polyunsaturated | Trans Fat |
|---|---|---|---|---|
| Safflower Oil | 0.8 | 10.2 | 2.0 | 0.0 |
| Canola Oil | 0.9 | 8.2 | 4.1 | 0.0 |
| Flaxseed Oil | 1.3 | 2.5 | 10.2 | 0.0 |
| Sunflower Oil | 1.4 | 2.7 | 8.9 | 0.0 |
| Margarine (stick) | 1.6 | 4.2 | 2.4 | 3.0 |
| Corn Oil | 1.7 | 3.3 | 8.0 | 0.0 |
| Olive Oil | 1.8 | 10.0 | 1.2 | 0.0 |
| Sesame Oil | 1.9 | 5.4 | 5.6 | 0.0 |
| Soybean Oil | 2.0 | 3.2 | 7.8 | 0.0 |
| Margarine (tub) | 2.0 | 5.2 | 3.8 | 0.5 |
| Peanut Oil | 2.3 | 6.2 | 4.3 | 0.0 |
| Cottonseed Oil | 3.5 | 2.4 | 7.0 | 0.0 |
| Vegetable Shortening | 3.2 | 5.7 | 3.3 | 1.7 |
| Chicken Fat | 3.8 | 5.7 | 2.6 | 0.0 |
| Lard (pork fat) | 5.0 | 5.8 | 1.4 | 0.0 |
| Beef Tallow | 6.4 | 5.4 | 0.5 | 0.0 |
| Palm Oil | 6.7 | 5.0 | 1.2 | 0.0 |
| Butter | 7.2 | 3.3 | 0.5 | 0.0 |
| Cocoa Butter | 8.1 | 4.5 | 0.4 | 0.0 |
| Palm Kernel Oil | 11.1 | 1.6 | 0.2 | 0.0 |
| Coconut Oil | 11.8 | 0.8 | 0.2 | 0.0 |

In analyzing any of the particular fats above, look first at the percentage of saturated fat. Obviously, coconut fat is "way bad," while canola oil is the best and has half as much saturated fat as olive oil. Monounsaturated fat is the most desirable of the three ingredients, For this, olive oil is the best—and again, coconut oil is the loser.

Make sure to watch out for the saturated fat in cheese. That is the big drawback of cheese, not to mention that it is a calorie-dense food. In 1909, according to records from the US Department of Agriculture, American meat intake was 123.9 pounds per person per year. Over the next century, meat intake soared, peaking at over 201.5 pounds per person per year in 2004. In the same interval, per-capita cheese intake rose from less than 4 pounds per year to nearly 34 pounds. The point is, eat as little cheese as possible.

---

[157] http://culinaryarts.about.com/od/culinaryreference/a/fattable.htm

# CARBOHYDRATES AND THE GLYCEMIC INDEX

Nutrients with calories fall into one of three categories: carbohydrates, fats, or proteins. In this chapter, we will take a close look at carbohydrates.

Under the classification of carbohydrates, a functional classification is that of simple carbohydrates or complex carbohydrates. In general, the simple sugars consist of monosaccharides and disaccharides, smaller (lower molecular weight) carbohydrates commonly referred to as "sugars." Examples of simple sugars are glucose, fructose, maltose, and sucrose. Because of their chemical structure, they absorb more quickly into the circulation, causing a rapid blood sugar elevation and the accompanying production of insulin. \

When we eat complex carbohydrates—those whose chemistry causes their molecules to be more tightly bound—they are more slowly absorbed. Grains, potatoes, and pasta are examples of complex carbohydrates.

**Enter the Glycemic Index**

A number system that tells us how fast a carbohydrate is absorbed into the bloodstream. Scientists have evaluated different carbohydrates and compared them to glucose to give us a number and thus the idea of a specific absorptive rate of any particular food. Scientists who measure glycemic index do so by giving 50 grams of a particular food to a subject and measuring the ensuing glucose response, then comparing it to the response from 50 grams of glucose. For example, if a particular food measures 70 percent compared to glucose, then its glycemic index is 70.

Glucose, the simple sugar, has a value of 100. Glucose is the food that all other carbohydrates are compared to. Complex carbohydrates, such as white bread (glycemic index 70) and white potatoes (glycemic index 85), are absorbed surprisingly rapidly, as shown by their higher glycemic index number. Note that some popular cereals have high glycemic indices, such as corn Flakes, Cheerios, and Bran Flakes, all with values around 90.

The glycemic index of our foods is consistently high, and why is that? Processing of our foods and the flour we use are the main reasons. So that foods will maintain a long shelf life, the flour in them is dramatically processed by removing the outer shell or husk of the grain, and likewise, the inner core is removed. The lost outer shell of the seed (bran) contains antioxidants, B vitamins, and fiber. The lost inner core (germ)—the "baby" of the seed, which grows into a new plant when pollinated—contains many vitamins, protein, minerals, and healthy fats. All of these things are removed in processed white flour.

Nutrient-rich, stone-ground flour has become a thing of past. A brief list of foods made with processed flour includes white bread, pastries, cakes, cookies, donuts, breakfast cereals, and pizza. A general principle, and a guiding light for you, is to know that the more the food is processed, the higher the glycemic index.

Unprocessed grains, on the other hand, contain significant amounts of fiber, which slows down the absorption of food. Some types of fiber are better than others. Fiber found in processed white bread or wheat flour has little effect in retarding the absorption of carbohydrates. The more viscous fiber found in whole oats and legumes does a better job in slowing the absorption of carbohydrates.

The glycemic index of natural sugars varies greatly. For instance, fructose (fruit sugar) has a glycemic index of 19, table sugar 61, honey 55, lactose (milk sugar) 46, maltose 105. Equally important to the glycemic index is the amount of carbohydrates a food has. Carrots have a fairly high glycemic index but few calories, so no problem. A baked potato has both a high glycemic index and a high calorie load, so the delivery of the carbohydrate to the body is high.

Research tells us that food with a higher glycemic index adversely affects cholesterol and insulin production and may cause cancer. Also, high glycemic index carbohydrates do not satisfy our hunger for as long. A glycemic index study was done on two groups of young boys. Both groups were given the same amount of calories for breakfast and lunch, but in one group the selection was from a low glycemic index source, and the other a high glycemic selection. Following lunch, and for a five-hour period, the boys were allowed to select any food they wanted that was available. The boys who were on the high-glycemic diet ate over 80 percent more calories than the boys who ate the low glycemic meals when allowed to graze at will.

When one is dieting to lose weight, glycemic index must be taken into consideration. The inability to stay the course and keep to a low-calorie diet is tied to glycemic index. The more simple carbohydrates a food contains, the more it is processed, the higher the glycemic index, the less likely a person can lose weight by eating it. Care must be taken not to judge a food solely on its glycemic index. Glycemic index is just another aid in selecting different foods affecting your health.

**Glycemic Index**

| | |
|---|---|
| Sucrose (table sugar) | 65 |
| Fructose (fruit sugar) | 25[158] |
| Lactose (milk sugar) | 46 |
| *Maltose | 105 |
| Donut | 76 |
| Croissant | 67 |

---

[158] http://www.sugar-and-sweetener-guide.com/glycemic-index-for-sweeteners.html

| | |
|---|---|
| Corn (sweet) | 54 |
| Carrots | 47 |
| Apple | 38 |
| Orange | 42 |
| Bean (kidney) | 28 |
| Bread (white) | 72 |
| Potato (mashed) | 92 |
| Bread (100 percent whole grain) | 51 |
| Rice | 110 |
| Cola | 97[159] |

*Maltose produced by allowing grain to soften in water and germinate. It is found in beverages, beer, cereal, pasta, potatoes, and many other processed products that have been sweetened.*

For a more complete list of foods and the glycemic index, Harvard Medical School has a wonderful online resource: http://www.health.harvard.edu/newsweek/Glycemic_index_and_glycemic_load_f or_100_foods.htm.

BOTTOM LINE: Avoid the five whites: white flour, white pasta, white rice, white potatoes, and sugar. Keep your eye on the fiber content of foods; the higher the fiber, the slower will be the absorption of carbohydrates into your system.

---

[159] http://www.health.harvard.edu/newsweek/Glycemic_index_and_glycemic_load_for_100_foods.htm

# PROTEIN, BEST SOURCES

If you aren't into a strict plant-based diet, then the following information will provide good guidelines for you to follow.

### Seafood twice weekly
Eat fish twice a week. The federal government's dietary guidelines (2011) recommend eight ounces of fish a week, providing 250 mg. of eicosapentaenoic acid (EPA) and docosahexaenoic acid (DHA), two main types of omega-3s. Listed below are some popular types of fish and the approximate total content of these two fatty acids in four-ounce portions of each:

Anchovies: 2,300-2,400 mg.
Cod: 200 mg.
Salmon (Atlantic, Chinook, Coho): 1,200-2,400 mg.
Sardines: 1,100-1,600 mg.
Scallops: 200 mg.
Trout: 1,000-1,100 mg.
Tilapia: 150 mg.
Yellowfin tuna: 150-350; canned: 150-300 mg.

### Meat and poultry, low-fat
Eat red meat sparingly. Let me say it again: *eat red meat sparingly.* On those rare occasions, choose lean or low fat . If you select ground beef, make sure it is at least 90 percent lean. Cut off excess fat and remove the skin from poultry.

### Eggs
An egg a day doesn't increase your cardiovascular risks. The yolk contains the saturated fat and cholesterol, so egg whites in particular can be eaten with impunity.

### Plant-based proteins
Plant-based proteins are better for you than animal-based proteins. Select legumes such as beans (kidney, pinto, black, split pea, chickpea), peas, and lentils. With about 30 percent of their calories coming from protein, lentils have the third-highest level of protein, by weight, of any legume or nut.

### Nuts
Nuts are a good source of omega-3s. Some nuts have more heart-healthy

nutrients and fats than others. Walnuts, almonds, and hazelnuts are good nuts to stick with. Cashews have more saturated fat, so best stay away from them. Peanuts have more protein than any of the other nuts. Almonds and pistachios both come in second. A one-ounce serving of most nuts contains two to three grams of fiber, the exception being cashews, which have just less than one gram of fiber per ounce. Fiber, as you know, is good. It also helps cut down the absorption of cholesterol from the gut.

# TRANS FAT

In 1902, Wilhelm Normann found that liquid oils could be hydrogenated to form trans fatty acids. These replaced beef tallow and tropical oils, which are very high in saturated fat. Trans fat became popular with consumers and food manufacturers because it acted as a preservative, giving foods a longer shelf life. It also gave foods a more tempting taste and texture.

The problem is, trans fat and excessive saturated fats are on the "forbidden list" of foods. In the May issue of *The American Journal of Clinical Nutrition*, Edmond K Kabagambe and colleagues reported on data from the study "Reasons for Geographical and Racial Differences in Stroke (REGARDS)," which studied more than 18,000 participants. "We suspected trans fat would increase the risk of death from multiple causes because some studies had already suggested that trans fat may increase occurrence of diseases such as cancer, diabetes and stroke. But we were surprised that the effect was actually quite large. Those who had the highest trans fat consumption had a 25 percent increased risk of death over the group with the lowest trans fat consumption."

At a seven-year follow-up study of the REGARDS participants, there were more than 1,500 deaths. It was found that people whose trans fatty acid consumption was as much as 3.5 to 4 percent of their daily energy intake had significantly higher rates of death from everything from stroke to diabetes to cancer.

"The implication, Kabagambe says, is the risk of death from major diseases could be reduced as much as 7 percent if trans fat were reduced to below 1 percent." So we definitely know that trans fat ingestion has a negative impact upon our health.[160]

Trans and saturated fats are ubiquitous in the foods we eat. A short list includes French fries, doughnuts, pizza, pastries, pie crusts, shortenings, and stick margarines. A small order of French fries has about three or four grams of trans fat. As you already know, when purchasing your food, looking at labels is always a wise thing to do. However, a food that claims zero percent trans fats could still have small amounts of trans fats because manufacturers are allowed to "round down" the figure. Any food with less than 0.5 grams per serving can claim 0.00 grams.

BOTTOM LINE: Be good about reading labels and noting the trans fat content. If it has trans fat, best leave it alone for the deleterious reasons shown by many well-designed studies.

---

[160] http://news.vanderbilt.edu/2013/04/study-reveals-broad-dangers-of-trans-fats/

# FIBER

Dietary fiber is important to a good diet and is beneficial for a number of reasons. First, it aids in providing fullness with and after meals. Second, adequate dietary fiber is associated with the reduction in cardiovascular disease, including peripheral arterial disease, high blood pressure, and hardening of the arteries. Third, it helps prevent constipation. Fourth, it helps keep blood sugar at normal levels. All of these are good things.

There are two types of fiber: soluble and insoluble. Soluble fiber attracts water, dissolves in water, and turns into a gel during digestion. It is readily fermented in the colon into gases and physiologically active byproducts. Most of the soluble fiber in vegetables and fruits are found in the skins and peels. When edible, always try to eat the whole vegetable or fruit.

Insoluble fiber does not dissolve in water and is found in foods such as wheat bran, vegetables, and whole grains. It adds bulk to the stool and appears to help food pass more quickly through the stomach and intestines.

Typically, the more refined or processed a food becomes, the lower its fiber content. Meals higher in fiber, besides being more healthy, are actually very tasty. As an example, for breakfast, try steel cut oats with nuts and berries instead of a plain, low-fiber, refined cereal. At lunch, have a sandwich on whole-grain bread and add vegetables, such as lettuce and tomato. With dinner, try brown rice or whole-grain noodles instead of white rice or pasta made with white flour. You can never go wrong with giving up white foods.

Psyllium, a common fiber supplement, is great, but consuming fiber from whole, natural foods is always the best choice. Here are a few whole foods that are high in natural fiber:

- ½ cup cooked black beans (7.5 grams)
- ½ medium avocado (5 grams)
- 1 cup cooked pearled barley (6 grams)
- 1 large pear with skin (7 grams)
- 1 cup fresh raspberries (8 grams)
- 1 ounce almonds (3.5 grams)

Most Americans consume inadequate amounts of fiber. Women should aim for 25 grams of fiber per day, while men should target 38 grams (or 21 and 30 grams daily, respectively, for those over the age of 51).

Note that when you consume fiber, you must also drink water to "puff up" the fiber. If you consume more than your usual intake of fiber but not enough fluid, you may experience side effects such as nausea or constipation. Boost your fiber intake slowly by adding two to three grams of fiber each week in order to prevent bloating, abdominal cramps, and stomach discomfort. Try to reach your fiber goal with whole foods so you get all the other benefits they provide. Learn how to read labels and count the grams of fiber in each food. It doesn't take long to get the required amount of fiber.

# WHOLE GRAINS

In this chapter, you will learn about whole grains, carbohydrates, and the glycemic Index. Not only is whole grain bread low in fat, but it is also a good source of B vitamins, vitamin E, magnesium, iron, and fiber, as well as other antioxidants. Whole grain bread releases its calories into the bloodstream more slowly, preventing a rapid rise of blood sugar. If you are a believer in the glycemic index, that is definitely a plus. This is not so important in an individual of healthy weight, but in the obese, pre-diabetic, and diabetic, a high glycemic index may lead to endothelial damage (lining of the vessels). Whole grains help retain cholesterol in the lumen of the bowel and encourage passage of "bad cholesterol" in the stool. Studies show that daily intake of two to three servings of whole grains a day leads to significant improvements in diabetes.

**Flour vs. Whole Grains**

Flour has a high glycemic index (a quick release of glucose); whole grains release glucose more slowly, avoiding spikes. Avoiding spikes is good, even if you don't have diabetes. Whole grains also have high levels of antioxidant activity. Antioxidants, of course, help slow the aging process.

There are many whole grains, but some of the more common are wheat, barley, oats, brown rice, quinoa, rye, millet, and buckwheat. In the rice family brown rice is best. The Harvard School of Public Health found that eating five or more servings of white rice per week resulted in an increased risk of type 2 diabetes. When the eating pattern changed to eating brown rice, the incidence of diabetes fell, and when going to other whole grains such as whole wheat and barley, the risk of type 2 diabetes went down even further.[161]

You saw the word "white" when rice was mentioned, didn't you? Restaurants seem to have an aversion to serving brown rice, and I suspect that's because white rice has a longer shelf life.

There are a couple of wheat flours that you need to know about because their inferiority to other grains in the nutritional scheme of things needs to be appreciated: bleached flour, all-purpose flour, and refined flour. Bleached and all-purpose flour is a blend of high-gluten hard wheat and low-gluten soft wheat, which makes it suitable for all baking and cooking needs. Bleaching is often done chemically; it also occurs naturally as flour ages. Refined white flour is flour from which the nutritious (and more perishable) bran and germ layers have been removed.

Rule: avoid foods with white flour. It is estimated that the average American

---

[161] http://www.hsph.harvard.edu/nutritionsource/diabetes-full-story/

consumes 17 to 22 slices of non-whole-grain bread per week. That is detrimental to good health. A breakfast of oatmeal or rolled oats would put a star on your forehead, particularly in lieu of cold cereal.

The good news is that under the Smarter Lunchrooms government program, our children are eating better. Besides low-fat dairy, vegetables, fruits, and lean meat, children are served whole grains. It is comforting to see better selection of foods for our posterity.

BOTTOM LINE: Choose whole grains when possible, and eat oatmeal for breakfast.

# RED MEAT, THINK AGAIN

What is red meat? Red meat, in traditional culinary terminology, is meat which is red when raw and not white when cooked. Red meat includes the meat of most adult mammals.

Red meat is high in saturated fats, and that is always bad. We also know that red meat is high in omega-6 fatty acids, which, when taken to excess, cause deleterious effects on various organs, particularly the heart.

The case against red meat began with a study conducted by Dr. Rashmi Sinha of the National Cancer Institute of more than 500,000 subjects. Sinha found that those who consumed four ounces of red meat daily were more than 30 percent likely to die within the next 10 years.[162] What does four ounces look like? It can fit in the palm of your hand—the size of a deck of cards. Processed meats such as bacon, sausage, hot dogs, and deli lunchmeats carry a higher risk of causing cancer than red meat.

The Harvard School of Public Health analyzed twenty studies involving more than 1.2 million people from 10 counties. The results showed that processed meats had, on average, four times more sodium and 50 percent more nitrate preservatives than unprocessed meats. Researchers found that eating just one serving of processed meat per day was associated with a 42 percent higher risk of heart disease and 19 percent higher risk of diabetes.[163]

Exposure to high concentrations of nitrosamines, carcinogenic compounds that can be produced from cooking meat at high temperatures, is associated with increased mortality from cancers of the esophagus, oral cavity, and pharynx. High cooking temperatures, like frying, can enhance the formation of nitrosamines. Simply put, the more you cook a meat, the more likely it will create carcinogens such as nitrosamines, a cancer-producing compound.

If, for whatever reason, you aren't impressed with these findings, red meat once or twice per month is a trade-off.

**Tips about Red Meat Consumption**

Try replacing minced red meat with minced Quorn (the leading meat-free brand within the UK and Ireland, available in the U.S. as well) or use lentils or beans instead. As an alternative to meat, eat more canned fish, including "the famous four": sardines, salmon, tuna, and mackerel. They are great in sandwiches or pasta dishes.

---

[162] http://www.washingtonpost.com/wp-dyn/content/article/2009/03/23/AR2009032301626.html

[163] http://www.valheart.com/blog/its-processed-meat-not-red-meat-that-harms-the-heart/

BOTTOM LINE: If you are into eating meat, aim for fish twice a week, and choosing chicken and turkey over beef, pork, lamb, or veal.

# MILK

I have selected a total of four milk products to compare in this chapter. However, because there are some minor variations from brand to brand and from store to store, the ingredients may not be exactly what you may find in your store, and the prices, likewise, will vary.

Mainly, let's look at comparisons between almond milk and the three milk products mentioned. Almond milk has 50 percent more calcium than other milk products, less calories, some fiber, and no saturated fat. Its other benefit is a longer shelf life than milk. For these reasons, I prefer almond milk.

A serving size is one cup, or 240 ml, which is equivalent to 8 ounces.

|  | Silk Almond Original | Organic Kirkland (1% low fat) | 1% low fat | 2% low fat |
|---|---|---|---|---|
| Calories | 60 | 130 | 120 | 140 |
| Total fat | 2.5 grams | 3 grams | 5 grams | 5 grams |
| Sodium | 160 mg | 160 mg | 120 mg | 125 mg |
| Carbs | 8 grams | 15 grams | 11 grams | 12 grams |
| Fiber | 1 gram | 0% | 0% | 0% |
| Sugar | 7 grams | 15 grams | 11 grams | 12 grams |
| Sat fat | 0 | 2 grams | 3 grams | 3 grams |
| Price | 4.1 cents / oz. | 5.6 cents / oz. | 1.54 cents / oz. | 1.54 cents / oz. |

# SALT

Salt has a very intriguing history. Some of the earliest evidence of salt extraction goes back around 6,000 years, when people living in Romania boiled spring water to extract the salt. In the days of the ancient Hebrews, Romans, and others, the presence or lack of salt caused conflict and was the source of many disputes and wars. Not only do we ingest salt, but it is used in religious ceremonies and has significance for many cultures. Salt has been used for centuries to preserve food.

Let's get a little more practical and ask ourselves, who consumes too much salt? Well, 90 percent of us do, at least in the U.S. I say "us," because I am one of the perpetrators, sorry to say. But I intend on changing that!

The CDC tells us that the average American consumes 3,400 milligrams per day of salt, and I have heard higher figures elsewhere. The U.S. Department of Health and Human Services recommends that higher-risk groups, such as those with cardiovascular disease, hypertension, diabetes, or chronic kidney disease limit sodium intake to 1,500 mg daily. The USDA recommends we all consume less than 2,300 mg per day each.[164] Take your pick of the numbers. In normal individuals free of comordid disease, I suggest using the 2,300 figure as the maximum.

High blood pressure is the number one risk factor for death in U.S. Children with a high-sodium diet have twice the chance of developing high blood pressure versus children with low-sodium diets.

Excess intake of salt may put you at risk for a number of disease processes. Add to the short list above heart failure, stroke, kidney stones, stomach cancer, and osteoporosis.

Excessive salt consumption is a key determinant of health and the largest determinant of preventable mortality worldwide. As *SFGate* recently reported, "Most studies agree that excessive consumption of salt increases the risk of cardiovascular disease. A study by scientists at the Federico II University of Naples Medical School published in November 2009 in 'BMJ' found that high salt intake increases the risk of cardiovascular disease and stroke." [165]

If you have high blood pressure, reducing your salt by about one-half teaspoon per day could drop your blood pressure by about two points.

**Ways to Cut Back on Salt**

---

[164] http://www.cnpp.usda.gov/Publications/NutritionInsights/insight3.pdf
[165] http://healthyeating.sfgate.com/side-effects-much-salt-intake-6577.html

1. Avoid or cut back on canned or processed food. Most of the salt you eat doesn't come from the saltshaker—it comes from processed foods in your diet. One can of soup has 1000 mg of salt. Rinse canned foods to remove some of the salt.
2. Buy fresh, plain frozen, or canned "no salt added" food. Substitute spices, herbs, and salt-free seasoning in cooking.
3. Cook rice, pasta, and hot cereal without salt. Cut back on instant or flavored mixes.
4. Cut back on prepared meals such as frozen dinners, pizza, and canned soups. You get the idea—anything out of a can is suspect.
5. If you're hooked on ready-to-eat breakfast cereals, choose cereals with low salt (sodium).
6. Put Elmer's glue on the bottom of your saltshaker. Taste before salting—your food that is.

## Salt Facts

1. Regular salt 1 tsp. = 2,360 mg of sodium
2. Sea Salt has the same amount of sodium as regular salt
3. Morton's salt substitute has no sodium
4. Low-sodium tamari (100% soy), 1 tsp. = 700 mg of sodium
5. South River Sweet White Miso, 1 tsp. = 115 mg of sodium
6. Kosher salt has half as much sodium as regular salt

# SUPPLEMENTS

Even in the face of the growing evidence that vitamins and mineral supplements do not affect illness, we in the U.S. spend about $12 billion a year on them. Their use has been primarily touted to benefit those with chronic disease. My experience working with patients tells me that over half of adults take multivitamins on a regular basis. That included myself—until about two years ago, when research began to suggest the lack of evidence of possible benefits of supplementation.

Research published in the *Annals of Internal Medicine* in December 2013 found that long-term multivitamin supplementation does not provide cognitive benefits in men aged 65 years or older. Mike Mitka, MSJ reported in JAMA that "The U.S. Preventive Services Task Force (USPSTF) found limited evidence supporting any benefit from vitamin and mineral supplementation for the primary prevention of cancer or cardiovascular disease."

In an accompanying editorial, the authors wrote, "Although available evidence does not rule out small benefits or harms or large benefits or harms in a small subgroup of the population, we believe that the case is closed—supplementing the diet of well-nourished adults with (most) mineral or vitamin supplements has no clear benefit and might even be harmful. These vitamins should not be used for chronic disease prevention. Enough is enough." [166]

These findings could certainly result in a lot of bottles removed from the medicine cabinet.

Unfortunately, most folks believe that herbs, vitamins, and minerals are extracted from nature and therefore must be not only effective but safe. This can be a dangerous theory. There are often interactions between over-the-counter supplements and prescribed drugs, resulting in adverse, even dangerous effects. Additionally, liver and kidney disease can compound the likelihood of the danger of supplements. You might want to go to a couple of websites—www.consumerlab.com and www.naturalstandard.com—and see if the supplement you are taking is safe for you.

The ineffectiveness of supplementation in the general population also extends to other realms. High-dose oral multivitamins and minerals do not reduce cardiovascular events in patients who have had a heart attack and who are receiving standard medications. Vitamins A and E, once thought to positively affect heart disease, do nothing for this problem. Beta-carotene (a precursor to vitamin A) may even be dangerous in higher doses.

Of course, there are cases where known nutritional deficiencies exist, and they must be treated. Vegetarians, note that there are very few supplements found in animal foods that are not better supplied by a plant-based diet. There

---

[166] http://jama.jamanetwork.com/article.aspx?articleid=1820428

are four nutrients which animal-based foods have that plant foods do not have: cholesterol and vitamins A, D, and B12. Three are non-essential; B12 is more problematic. Plants grown in non-organic soil may be deficient in vitamin B12. So, vegans may need to supplement extra B12.

There you have it. Supplements are a waste of money. There is nothing more expensive than a medication that does not work.

BOTTOM LINE: All our vitamins and minerals can be found in a well-rounded nutritious diet to supply our physiological needs.

# ASPIRIN

So much is said about aspirin, so much aspirin around we are almost bathed in it. How many people in America have taken an aspirin in the last 24 hours? I don' know, but I suspect a lot. The Aspirin Foundation tells us that aspirin, one of the first drugs to come into common usage, is still the most widely used medication in the world, with approximately 35,000 metric tons consumed annually.[167] That translates into over 100 billion aspirin tablets every year.

What is this ubiquitous compound with such wide acclaim? Chemically it is *acetylsalicylic acid*. The father of modern medicine, Hippocrates (c. 460 - c. 377 BC), used a powder made from the bark and leaves of the willow tree. This may have been the beginning of the aspirin legacy. In our modern era, the active ingredient of aspirin was first discovered in the bark of the willow tree by Edward Stone in 1763. A French chemist, Charles Frederic Gerhardt, was the first to prepare acetylsalicylic acid in 1853.

In 1897, chemists working at Bayer AG, a company in Germany, produced a synthetically altered version of salicin. The new drug, formally acetylsalicylic acid, was called *aspirin* by Bayer AG after the old botanical name for meadowsweet, *Spiraea ulmaria*. By 1899, Bayer had worldwide distribution of its new drug, and the popularity of aspirin grew over the first half of the 20th century. Bayer's patent expired way back in 1917, and the sales of Bayer Aspirin declined dramatically with the introduction of acetaminophen (Tylenol).

In addition to its analgesic properties, thirty-plus years ago, the anti-clotting effects of aspirin were discovered. And aspirin sales have now bounced back with the discovery of its ability to help prevent vascular complications such as heart attacks and strokes when taken preventatively in low doses. As reported in the *European Heart Journal* in 2013, an analysis of 16 secondary prevention trials in patients with previous heart attack, stroke, or transient cerebral attack (near-stroke) found an absolute reduction in the yearly incidence of non-fatal events of about 10 to 20 per 1,000 patients—and to a smaller, but still definite, reduction in vascular death.[168]

It is important to note the "previous heart attack" factor. This means those studied were proven to already have cardiovascular disease. We call this "secondary prevention," and clearly, there is a benefit to taking aspirin in this case.

Now let's talk about the cost/benefit ratio, as business folks would put it. The increase in gastrointestinal bleeding is present, but the benefits of anti-platelet (clot prevention) therapy substantially exceed the risks.

---

[167] http://www.aspirin-foundation.com
[168] http://eurheartj.oxfordjournals.org/content/current

As for primary prevention—preventing disease, or the *sequelae* (condition) of a disease before it happens—let's take a look. An overview of nine studies published in *European Heart Journal* in 2013 showed that out of 254 patients without existing cardiovascular disease who took aspirin daily for seven years, only one person was prevented from having a cardiovascular event, and in that same pool, one person could be expected to have a major bleeding episode as a result.[169]

Seems aspirin may not have a role in of primary prevention.

BOTTOM LINE: If you do not now have cardiovascular disease and are tempted to take aspirin to prevent that stroke or heart attack, check with your doctor first, as your individual health profile, your current medication list, and other risk factors will all come into play as factors in your decision.

---

[169] http://eurheartj.oxfordjournals.org/content/34/44.toc

# CURCUMIN, FOUND IN CURRY

*Curcumin*, the principal chemical in the vivid yellow spice turmeric (*Curcuma longa*), is thought to have antioxidant properties that blunt the effects of aging. Curcumin can overpower pro-inflammatory proteins called *cytokines*, and that is good news. It's being explored as a cancer treatment in part because inflammation appears to play a role in cancer.

According to the *Journal of the American Medical Association*, a constituent of turmeric might also have potential for treating cystic fibrosis. Scientists in the United States and Canada are using the substance to correct the defect in mice with a form of cystic fibrosis.[170]

Bharat B. Aggarwal, PhD, a professor at the University of Texas MD Anderson Cancer Center and the author of *Healing Spices,* tells us that curcumin is "50 times more potent than vitamin C or E" as an antioxidant.[171] (See the section on Antioxidants.) One study showed that curcumin inhibits the growth of certain breast cancer cells, and other research suggests it may also protect against stomach and colon cancer.

In 2013, *Audio Digest* reported that curcumin, long-cultivated in Asia for culinary and medical purposes, might also have potential as a chemopreventative agent for colorectal and pancreatic cancers. In order to absorb adequately, it must be given in a high dose or in conjunction with black pepper (whose active ingredient is piperine), which increases the absorption of curcumin a thousand-fold.[172]

Curcumin may also be of use in treating Alzheimer's disease. According to an article published by the National Institutes of Health, the prevalence of Alzheimer's among adults aged 70 to 79 in India, where turmeric is a very common part of the diet, is 4.4 times less than that of adults in the same age bracket in the U.S. And researchers who studied a group of Asian elders between 60 and 93 found that those who ate curry (containing turmeric, which is often found in curry) "occasionally" or "very often" had significantly better cognitive scores than those who "never or rarely" consumed curry.[173]

A disclaimer: curcumin is said to interact with certain drugs such as blood thinning agents, ibuprofen, and ibuprofen-like drugs and is not recommended for persons with biliary tract obstruction, because it stimulates bile secretion.

In case you didn't know, curries can be made with a variety of spices, but, turmeric (containing curcumin) is often found in most curry powders and pastes.

---

[170] http://jama.jamanetwork.com/article.aspx?articleid=198769

[171] *Healing Spices: How to Use 50 Everyday and Exotic Spices to Boost Health and Beat Disease*, Bharat B. Aggarwal PhD and Debora Yost, Sterling, January 2011

[172] http://www.audio-digest.org/editorial/meetings/MSEPS2013.pdf

[173] http://www.ncbi.nlm.nih.gov/pmc/articles/PMC2781139/

In the Western world, curry powder mixtures tend to have a fairly standardized taste, though a great variety of spice mixtures are used in Indian cuisine. Because curries are all different, it's challenging to offer precise generic nutritional data, but here is what the USDA has to say about one tablespoon of curry powder:

Calories : 20 kcal
Fat: 1 g
Carbohydrates: 4 g
Fibers: 2 g
Protein: 1 g[174]

Curry powder is delicious, but a report in *Nutrition and Cancer* 55(2), 126–131 showed that pure turmeric powder has the highest curcumin concentration. Depending on the brand, curcumin content varies from one batch of turmeric powder to another, but the percentage has been estimated to be between 1.06 percent and 5.70 percent in the brands tested.[175] As always read labels.

[174] http://nutritiondata.self.com/facts/spices-and-herbs/185/2
[175] http://li123-4.members.linode.com/files/Curcumin%20Content%20of%20Turmeric%20and%20Curry%20Powders_0.pdf

# EXERCISE, SHEEHAN THE MENTOR

Sometime around 1975, I met Dr. George Sheehan in a small amphitheater at the University of Utah while he was giving a lecture on running. I was impressed and enlightened. So when my wife asked me to "jog" with her, I took her up on it. She had already been doing it for several weeks, so when we hit the asphalt outside our home, she slowed down while I did the scout pace. You remember the scout pace, I am sure: run 50 steps, walk 50 steps.

After a couple of weeks, I could jog without stopping, though only for about one mile. My wife was very tolerant of my snail-like speed. Wasn't long until I convinced two of my friends to join me in this newfound life of running. Within a year, we contemplated running a marathon. Our little group of three trained, with Monday nights being our "long run." We would run seven and a half miles up to Sugar House Park and seven and a half miles back home.

Before a plantar fascial injury terminated my marathon career, I had run 10 marathons, with each successive marathon time better than the one before. I never won a race, but I always finished.

Dr. Sheehan was both a philosopher and a runner, and I liked that combination. The oldest of 14 children, he had followed in the footsteps of his father and become a cardiologist. He and his wife raised 12 children. He had been a track star at Manhattan College, so when he took up running again mid-life, it was not a new concept. He renewed his "running license" and also went back to being a philosopher. He read The Greeks, Thoreau, Emerson, and James, among other philosophical works. It was what Ireneus, one of the early Catholic fathers, said that caught his attention: "The glory of God is man fully functioning." Sheehan took that to mean *physically* as well in other areas where he felt fulfilled, such as his professional and family life.

With this goal in mind, nothing would hold him back or slow him down. He began in with backyard running loops. There were 26 loops to a mile. Once that became boring, he ran the river road on his lunch hour. Within five years, he ran a 4:47 mile, which was the world's first sub-five-minute time by a 50-year-old. He then began writing a weekly column in the local paper and eventually became a national fitness expert. His intriguing personality made him not only believable but also respected and sought after.

Sheehan wrote his newspaper column for 25 years. He was also the medical editor for *Runner's World Magazine* and lectured around the world. Unfortunately, he developed prostate cancer in 1986 and, since it had already spread to his skeletal system, it took his life seven years later. Once he began to anticipate a shorter life span, the tenor of his articles and talks changed. He continued to search for the truths of life—his time not about running, but about dying. "We are all unique, never-to-be-repeated events," he said. He wanted to leave nothing on the court at his death.

One of his favorite quotes was from Robert Frost: "I am no longer concerned with good and evil. What concerns me is whether my offering will be acceptable."

I remember Sheehan the most for his philosophy about aging. He was in touch with the ever-changing challenges and opportunities of growing older. He continued to run, and he continued to tell about life's beauties, no matter the stumbling blocks, no matter the number of birthdays. His life is an example of never being too old to go after your dreams.

Sheehan records, "No sense in dwelling on the past or wondering about the future. I have to resist the tendency that comes with age; I cannot waste my time on memories of the past—being old is different from being middle-aged is being single is from being married. Many who enter this stage dislike it. We cannot presume that success in one stage of life will be repeated in the next."[176]

I myself have noticed that every decade has a different set of challenges, needing a different set of answers. Perhaps the questions pile up faster than the answers do. Some people just seem to be able to accelerate into the next year, the next decade, the next challenge. We may enter into the next phase of life (or any phase) by just dipping a toe to test the water, but we eventually jump in, taking on the goal of swimming to the other side, rather than floating, just to keep our head above the water.

The next section of this book that you are about to embark on could be a bewildering experience, but I believe the chances of success are going to be greater than you have anticipated. This can only happen if you take the stance of "If it is going to be, it is up to me."

BOTTOM LINE: I found a mentor I wished to follow. Find yourself a mentor. I guarantee it will make a difference.

---

[176] http://www.georgesheehan.com/bio.html

# EXERCISE AND PHYSICAL ACTIVITY

One in ten deaths in the United States is associated with a sedentary lifestyle. Not unexpectedly, older individuals tend to be more physically inactive. It is logical to expect that chronic health conditions due to a sedentary lifestyle will increase.

Inactivity indeed accelerates the onset of chronic health conditions, not the least of which is physical frailty. Physical inactivity accounts for approximately 15 percent of the U.S. healthcare budget. In 1996, 83 percent of prescription drugs, 66 percent of physician visits, and 55 percent of emergency department visits were made by persons with chronic health conditions. In hospital admissions, chronic health problems existed in 69 percent of those admitted—the length of stay in the hospital almost doubled in the same population.[177] It is estimated that widespread practice of regular, moderate physical activity would shave approximately $119 billion yearly from the healthcare budget.[178]

It is interesting to take a look at the leading causes of death over these last 100 years. The leading cause of death in 1900 was from infection, shifting now to tobacco use, obesity, and physical inactivity. If by now you aren't getting the message of where we are in this country and where we should be, then it's going to take divine intervention to make the connection.

Let's take a look where it all begins. According to the Institute of Medicine (IOM), some children may receive physical education only once per week or not at all.[179] Physical exercise/activity remains an important part of maintaining health throughout life. We find that fewer than half of U.S. youth get at least 60 minutes of moderate or vigorous activity each day, as recommended by the Department of Health and Human Services Physical Activity folks.[180]

This isn't the way to get one of the most important lifestyle areas ingrained into our culture. We have to take care of our young people and not teach them that physical activity is secondary to just about everything else. IOM panel member Charles H. Hillman, PhD, said there is a growing body of literature suggesting that physical activity promotes cognitive health by promoting beneficial changes in the brain that may support attention and memory.[181] Children simply perform better after physical activity.

---

[177] *United States Health Care and the Future Supply of Physicians,* Eli Ginzberg and Panos Minogiannis, Transaction Publishers; 1 edition (November 1, 2003)

[178] http://www.ncbi.nlm.nih.gov/books/NBK83160/

[179] http://jama.jamanetwork.com/article.aspx?articleid=1710452

[180] http://www.cdc.gov/mmwr/preview/mmwrhtml/rr6005a1.htm

[181] http://jama.jamanetwork.com/article.aspx?articleid=1710453

We have an epidemic of physical inactivity. Forty to fifty million U.S. adults do not meet recommended physical activity levels. That is a heck of a lot of people!

But what is physical activity, anyway? Physical activity includes any activity that can be worked into your daily routine, such as taking the stairs at work, parking farther from the grocery store entrance, walking rather than riding, and so forth. The key word is "move."

The other consideration is exercise. Back to the interrogation. What is exercise? Every word has a particular meaning. *Exercise* means following a constructed plan of physical activity that is well-formulated and followed regularly, and causes a cardiovascular workload, with a goal of self-improvement. The goal is a well-formulated program which is regularly applied and gets your heart rate to a point of physiological benefit. That is a big load to dump on you!

Bear with me a moment, as I want to place obesity and sedentary lifestyle side by side. Most people believe that the number one failure of our American lifestyle is overeating. The statistics in Utah are better than most states. In Utah, in the year 2012, 24.3 percent of the adult population was obese—not just overweight, but obese, meaning that their body mass index (BMI) was 30 or more.[182] Half of all adults in the U.S. will be obese by 2030, according to an article in Lancet.[183]

According to the World Health Organization, non-communicable diseases kill more than 36 million people each year. Physical inactivity accounts for 6 percent of these deaths—a higher figure than the 5 percent attributed to overweight and obesity issues.[184] Yet there is more excitement in the medical community about "fat America."

The reality is, fitness matters more than fatness. Underline that sentence with your yellow marker! Where are the advocates for physical fitness? Statistics tell us that 41 percent of patients have never had their doctor talk to them about physical exercise or physical fitness—no, never.

Lack of fitness is part of our culture, starting from a very young age. Research tells us that only 5 percent of all children, kindergarten to high school graduation, are offered a physical activity opportunity in their school. That isn't the way I remember it when I went to school. "No child left behind," should be "No child with a big behind!" That slogan didn't begin with me, but I strongly subscribe to the concept.

A study published in January 2014 in *European Heart Journal* of 743,497 Swedish men showed that fit teenagers can reduce the likelihood of a heart attack in later life. The subjects were followed from age 18 for an average of 34 years. Forty-three percent of the study participants were at normal weight

---

[182] http://www.fasinfat.org/states/ut/

[183] http://www.washingtonpost.com/national/health-science/half-of-us-adults-will-be-obese-by-2030-report-says/2011/08/25/gIQAYthweJ_story.html

[184] http://www.who.int/mediacentre/factsheets/fs355/en/

during their teens and were determined to be physically fit. Fitness was determined by the use of a stress test done on a bicycle. Additionally, men who were obese but fit in their teen-age years had a higher risk of developing a heart attack than if they were lean but unfit.

They concluded that every 15 percent increase in fitness level decreased the risk of developing a heart attack 30 years later by 18 percent. Those who regularly pursued fitness in their late teenage years reduced the risk of a premature heart attack by 35 percent.[185]

In analyzing this whole package of physical activity, researchers found that the most predictive feature of getting patients to become fit was for the MD to be a model. In other words, patients were highly swayed by their doctors' personal fitness routines.

Just to get our arms around physical fitness, those who research all this lifestyle intervention stuff suggest we do 150 minutes weekly of moderate exercise. How many days a week do you perform moderate intensity physical activity? Moderate exercise means increasing both your breathing rate and heart rate above normal values. There is a more technical definition, but that won't be part of this discussion. The higher the heart rate, the more cardiovascular benefit there will be. Of course, there is an upper limit, which won't concern 95 percent of the adult population.

Walking is good, biking is good, swimming is good, treadmill is good—just to mention some of the most popular modes of exercise. Hippocrates said, "Walking is man's best friend." You might consider the other man's best friend, the dog, and let him take you for a walk. If you have an infant or small child, push or jog with your stroller.

BOTTOM LINE: Get your whole family involved. You know the way you should be living. Be the leader in your family… and why not also recruit your friends to be a part of a better and healthier life through exercise?

---

[185] http://www.irishcentral.com/opinion/others/fitness-in-early-adulthood-reduces-chances-for-heart-attacks-239814671-240124861.html

# EXERCISE PRESCRIPTION

Paramount to the prevention of having an unhealthful weight problem and, for that matter, treating the weight problem, is the idea of a routine, well-thought-out, and well-executed physical activity program. The federal guidelines of 2008 recommend at least 150 minutes a week of moderate-intensity aerobic physical activity.[186] The Institute of Medicine, on the other hand, suggests 60 minutes a day as an optimal activity goal for patients.[187]

Being successful at an exercise program requires that you consider four areas:

1. type of exercise
2. intensity
3. duration
4. frequency

Let's look into each.

**Type of Exercise:** Any exercise that engages large muscle groups, such as the legs, in rhythmic movements for a sustained time period is appropriate. For example, brisk walking, jogging, hiking, cycling, swimming, cross-country skiing, and skating. The more enjoyable the exercise, the more likely you will stick with it, so choice is important. The problem comes when you're not excited about any exercise.

**Intensity:** Beginners should start at an intensity perceived as "mildly difficult," which generally translates to a heart rate range of 55 to 65 percent of their maximum heart rate. To figure out your maximum heart rate, take your age and subtract it from 220. So, if you are 40 years old, your maximum heart rate is 180. Then, multiply that number by .6 (for 60 percent, which splits the difference between 55 and 65 percent). Your goal heart rate is 108 beats per minute.

That is very doable, initially. Looking forward, as you become better conditioned, you can increase your goal to 70 to 80 percent of your heart rate. Caution: You should always consult your doctor before beginning a new physical exercise routine. And make sure you work up to the higher rate slowly and over a period of days to weeks.

**Duration:** Exercising for 30 to 40 minutes at a time is recommended to achieve and maintain fitness. However, always start with less time and effort,

---

[186] http://www.cdc.gov/physicalactivity/everyone/guidelines/adults.html

[187] http://www.iom.edu/Reports/2013/Educating-the-Student-Body-Taking-Physical-Activity-and-Physical-Education-to-School.aspx

then work up. Any time chest pain, jaw pain, or arm pain occurs while exercising, stop and get medical help. If you have chosen walking as your preferred form of exercise, as most people do, an initial goal of 10 miles a week is reasonable. For example, walk two miles a day, five days a week.

**Frequency:** Having now determined the type of exercise, intensity, and duration just right for you, the last thing to figure out is how often you will do it. You may, depending on age, weight, general mobility, and state of conditioning, want to start off with three times per week, eventually hoping to work up to five or six times a week. There are some folks who like to break it up their physical activity into twice-a-day sessions. That is a personal preference.

All exercise sessions should include warm-ups and stretching. Your rate of progression will depend on your age, health status, and functional capacity. Most sedentary adults require an initial phase of four to six weeks during which the training sessions are structured to minimize discomfort, and both duration and intensity are kept at a low level. This is often a critical period, since a bad experience at the onset may be detrimental to long-term adherence.

During the next phase (two to three months), the major physiologic adaptations to exercise begin. Increases in intensity and duration can occur every few weeks until the exercise program is compatible with your overall training goals. For older and higher-risk persons, the progression should be slower.

This won't be overwhelming news, but different activities burn up a different number of calories. These can be measured in METs, or metabolic equivalents. The MET concept represents a simple, practical, and easily understood procedure for expressing the energy cost of physical activities. One MET is defined as the energy it takes to sit quietly. In each exercise session you want to be doing three to six METs.

Moderate intensity activities are those that get you moving fast enough or strenuously enough to burn off three to six times as much energy per minute as you do when you are sitting quietly. Brisk walking fits the bill for moderate-intensity activity. How fast is brisk? For the average person, it means walking four miles an hour, or about as fast as you'd walk if you were late for an important appointment.

In the table below, you will get an idea of which activity might be optimal for you.

**Energy Requirements of Common Daily Activities**

| LEISURE ACTIVITIES | METs |
|---|---|
| Mild | |
| Playing the piano | 2.3 |
| Canoeing (leisurely) | 2.5 |

| | |
|---|---|
| Golfing (with cart) | 2.5 |
| Walking (2 mph) | 2.5 |
| Ballroom dancing (slow) | 2.9 |
| **Moderate** | |
| Walking (3 mph) | 3.3 |
| Cycling (leisurely) | 3.5 |
| Calisthenics (no weight) | 4.0 |
| Golfing (no cart) | 4.4 |
| Swimming (slow) | 4.5 |
| Walking (4 mph) | 4.5 |
| **Vigorous** | |
| Chopping wood | 4.9 |
| Tennis (doubles) | 5.0 |
| Ballroom dancing (fast) or square dancing | 5.5 |
| Cycling (moderately) | 5.7 |
| Skiing (water or downhill) | 6.8 |
| Climbing hills (no load) | 6.9 |
| Swimming | 7.0 |
| Walking (5 mph) | 8.0 |
| Jogging (10 min mile) | 10.2 |
| Rope skipping | 12.0 |
| Squash | 12.1 |

*Journal of the American Heart Association* reported on a study, done at the prestigious Cooper Clinic in Dallas, TX, between 1970 and 1983, which showed that a 1-MET increase in low-risk patients resulted in an 18 percent reduction in long-term cardiovascular mortality such as heart attack deaths.[188] Men and women thirty to fifty years of age participated in the study. Looking at the chart above would tell us it doesn't take much to get up to more than 1 Met. Not surprisingly, highly fit individuals achieve the greatest protection.

The investigators of the Cooper Clinic study reported, "Our data is of additional importance, given that a 1-MET increase was associated with reductions in 30-year mortality rate, a potentially more informative end point for low-risk individuals in midlife."[189] This is a fairly select group in that they started with low-risk individuals. It doesn't take much of a leap of faith to realize that for the person who is sedentary, the benefits would be greater.

Message: the higher the MET, the longer you live.

BOTTOM LINE: Depending upon your age, any health issues you already have (like high blood pressure, diabetes, etc.), and whether you intend to incorporate a

---

[188] http://circ.ahajournals.org/content/125/1/e2.full

[189] http://jaha.ahajournals.org/content/1/4/e001354.full

moderate to high-intensity exercise program, consider checking with your physician first. In constructing your exercise program, apply the prescription of type, intensity, duration, and frequency.

# THE WALKING STORIES

Thomas Jefferson said, "The sovereign invigorator of the body is exercise, and of all the exercises walking is the best." Though he didn't know it, he was talking about brain neurotransmitters, primarily endorphins. Endorphins are produced by the pituitary gland and the hypothalamus during exercise. These, as well as other neuroactive chemicals, lead to good mental health.

In a 1990 meta-analysis summarizing eighty studies of exercise and depression, a research team that included psychologist Penny McCullagh, PhD reported that exercise was a beneficial antidepressant both immediately and over the long term.[190] Exercise was an equally effective antidepressant for both genders. The greater the length of the exercise program and the larger the total number of exercise sessions, the greater the decrease in depression with exercise. Walking and jogging were the most frequent forms of exercise researched.

Beyond the limited boring physiology just described, great things occur within the mind when walking. Nietzsche, German philosopher of the late 19th century, tells us, "All truly great thoughts are conceived while walking." Maybe just being alone with your thoughts and away from the many external buffetings of the pounding waves of life is what it is all about.

George Will felt this way about walking: "Walking is the most civil and civilizing exercise, because it is the one most conducive to thinking." Who can knock thinking nowadays, when thinking is unrealistic and cumbersome, because it may slow us down.

Charles Dickens was a promiscuous walker through London both day and night. It was reported that he would take 20-mile walks to quiet or exhaust his restless energy. Walking at a quick pace invigorates the cardiovascular system, yet gives us enough time to look in front of us to see the flowers, or count the trees as we pass, or even watch insects as they go about their meaningful existence.

The walk that has held my attention since I learned of it was the 22-mile walk from Alpine, Utah to the Salt Lake Temple. John R. Moyle was born in England in the early 1800s but lived in Alpine later in his life. During the construction of the temple, he was the chief superintendent of masonry. Because he needed to be onsite by 8 a.m. on Monday morning, John would start walking about 2 a.m. in order to cover the 22 miles. He would stay onsite all week, then on Friday, he would set out walking south to his home at 5 p.m. to be with his family in Alpine for the weekend, arriving there shortly before midnight.

---

[190] *Why Not Stay Fat? - Overweight? So What. 'Be Happy with Who and What You Are',* Wayne Lambert,

Then, tragedy struck him—literally. Only a few of us now remember how unpredictable the milking of a cow can go. One of his cows struck out during milking and kicked John Moyle in the leg, shattering the bone just below the knee. This was in a rural area, and medical help was scarce and inadequate at best. A bucksaw that had been used to cut branches from a nearby tree was used to amputate his lower leg just a few inches below the knee.

Not one to shirk his commitment, Moyle took a piece of wood and carved himself an artificial leg. He tested the device on his healing limb, then, as he became stronger and more confident, resumed his capacity as a stonecutter. When he felt he could stand the pain, he strapped on his leg, then continued to walk the 22 miles to Salt Lake Temple.

BOTTOM LINE: Walking as an activity has monumental benefits, not always easy to measure.

# EXERCISE: THE 10-MILE WALKING PROGRAM

It may have been a long time since you were physically active. You might just be taking a break from a well-designed exercise program, or possibly you have been sedentary most of your adult life. No matter. You are the captain of your ship, and you give the orders. Waste no more time; grab the wheel!

When a captain of a ship sees he is off course, he wastes no time by expounding upon his mistake, but instead recalculates, changes course, steers purposefully toward his destination, and with renewed courage, makes up the time he has lost. Here is part of the map that you can refer to as you head for the security of the harbor.

## Benefits of Walking

- Lose, then maintain a normal weight
- Prevent and treat chronic diseases such as diabetes, heart disease, high blood pressure, and peripheral artery disease
- Strengthen your bones and decrease bone loss from aging
- Improve your mood
- Provide a venue for social contacts (group activity)
- Improve muscle strength, balance, and flexibility

When considering an exercise program, there are many things to work into the what, when, and how much. This 10-Mile Program keeps it simple for you. All I want you to do is walk 10 miles per week. Take a brisk walk each day, and you'll live a healthier life.

First, choose a time to do your walking. If you want, you can even break up your daily walk into two parts—one in the morning and one in the afternoon or early evening. Do your stretching for a few minutes, then begin your walk.

As a beginner, it is important that you always start out slow and walk a short distance at first. I suggest you walk a half-mile a day for one week, five days out of the seven. That first week, walk slowly. Then, walk one mile for one week, then one and a half miles for one week, then two miles the next week. If you get sore, stiff, or achy, walk for less distance for a longer period of time. Try to work up to walking two miles a day, five days a week.

Once you are securely in a routine of 10 miles a week, pick up your pace and try to cut 10 to 30 seconds off each mile. Eventually, you should end up with a fairly brisk walk, with your goal being to walk each mile in 15 minutes. Of course, circumstances and people being different, you may end up with a very brisk walk with less than a 15-minute mile, or a slower pace of 16 minutes or more.

Always be alert to chest pain, left arm pain, or jaw pain. This may indicate heart problems. If you experience any of these, or excess fatigue, see your doctor without delay.

If you follow the 10-Mile Program and walk five days a week regularly, you will soon have traveled more than 500 miles in a year. You will need new shoes! Speaking of your shoes, watch to see if the soles start to separate from the upper portion. If the heels, viewed from the back, wear excessively on either the inside or outside, or there is heel asymmetry when comparing the heels, purchase a new pair.

Walking speed matters less than distance and your weight. A good rule of thumb is 65 calories burned per-mile for a 120-pound person, 100 calories for a 180-pound person, 115 calories burned for a 200-pound person, and 140 calories burned for a 250-pound person.

# NON-EXERCISE ACTIVITY THERMOGENESIS

The three components of daily energy expenditure are:
1. Basal metabolic rate (just existing without exercise or activity), accounting for about 60 to 70 percent of daily caloric expenditure
2. Thermic effect of food (heat given off or calories burned in the breakdown of ingested food), accounting for about 10 percent of daily caloric expenditure
3. Activity thermogenesis (calories used in activity of daily living), including exercise and non-exercise activity thermogenesis (NEAT)

As we discussed in a previous chapter, NEAT is the burning of calories beyond simply existing in the awakened state. Non-exercise-related energy expenditure (NEAT) is pivotal in the regulation of human energy expenditure and body weight regulation.

Studies suggest that NEAT may differ by as much as 2,000 calories per day between two adults of similar size and weight, because of differing occupations and leisure-time activities. We also know that lean individuals tend naturally to be more active than obese or overweight individuals. Obese individuals, overall, stand and ambulate two and a half hours per day less than lean individuals.[191] That is something never to forget—it's really important.

Conversely, when obese or overweight people lose weight, their activity levels generally do not increase. These findings suggest that there is a genetic component to NEAT. This is not offered as an excuse, just a fact that may help us understand the difficulty in trying to losing weight.

What does all this mean and how can we use it to our advantage? We should provide patients with a choice of physical activities. Again, you are better able to choose what might work for you. The choice the patient makes will most likely insure that the activity will have higher compliance rate. We should recommend activities that have immediate rewards, such as walking while listening to music. Convenience of the activity also improves compliance. We should try to identify barriers to why the activity may never be engaged in or why it may fail after a short term of application.

You should make a list of what activities you are engaged in that prevent effective NEAT, such as watching too much TV or habitually taking the shortest distance from point A to point B when you need to get about. Then, list all the things that you can do to increase your NEAT, such as standing up rather than sitting, walking around a little more, taking the stairs once in a while, even doing things like hand-washing your dishes or getting out to do yard work more often.

---

[191] http://atvb.ahajournals.org/content/26/4/729.full

Choose walking rather than using your car, use stairs rather than taking the elevator, choose a more difficult walking path. I think you get the idea.

These are fairly pointed, impactful suggestions you have just read. I strongly urge you to get pencil and paper and do as instructed.

BOTTOM LINE: Anything but sitting or sleeping is NEAT, I mean, really neat. You're "neater" when you purposefully go out of your way to move that body. Think "move" in everything you do.

# U.S. DEPT. OF HEALTH AND HUMAN SERVICES EXERCISE RECOMMENDATIONS

The information about physical activity listed below, borrowed from the U.S. Department of Health and Human Services, is probably the most authoritative and complete in this whole book. It's a good summary for what you have already learned.

- Adults should strive to be physically active for at least two hours and 30 minutes each week (about 30 minutes per day, five days per week) at a moderate-to-vigorous level.
- Or, get at least one hour and 15 minutes of vigorous-intensity aerobic physical activity per week.
- Episodes of vigorous aerobic activity should be performed for a minimum of 10 minutes at a time, spread throughout the week.
- Increasing the intensity or the amount of time that you are physically active can have even greater health benefits and can help control body weight.
- 60 to 90 minutes per day can prevent or reverse weight gain.
- Adults should include muscle-strengthening activities that involve all muscle groups at least two times per week.
- Older adults (65 and older) should follow the guidelines for adults, but if this is not possible due to a chronic or medical condition, they should strive to be as physically active as their condition, and physician, allows.
- Older adults should avoid inactivity.
- Older adults should do exercises that maintain or improve balance.
- Children and adolescents (ages 6 to17) should be physically active for at least 60 minutes every day, or most every day.
- Activities should be at a moderate or vigorous intensity level. They should include muscle or bone-strengthening activities at least three days per week.
- Rather than emphasis on team sports, exercise should be about developing healthy lifestyle activities and habits.[192]

To avoid injury and reduce soreness, start slowly. Gradually build up to your goal while giving your body time to adjust. Furthermore, getting the recommended amount of physical activity does not mean spending money on a costly membership at the gym or expensive equipment for your home. However, professional help could be advantageous in getting you started in the right way.

Regular exercise reduces the risk of developing or dying from some of the

---

[192] http://www.health.gov/paguidelines/pdf/paguide.pdf

leading causes of death in the United States such as diabetes, colon cancer, heart disease and stroke, and high blood pressure. It helps promote well being, and is useful in the treatment of depression and anxiety.

# STAY ACTIVE, IMPROVE YOUR DIET, CONTINUE TO WORK

Japan can take pride in the life expectancy of citizens in their number one and number three prefectures. Recent events revealed that Okinawan women fell from the number one spot to number three in life expectancy, but another city in Japan got the honor of being number one in the whole world: Nagano.

Okinawa has been in first place since the statistics first were published in 1975. Okinawan women who were born in 2010 are expected to live to be 87.02 years old. But, nowadays, that isn't good enough to win the gold medal—that puts Okinawa women only in third place in the nation. Men's life expectancy in Okinawa also went down to 79.4 years, which puts them in 30th place in the nation.

A quick review notes that Okinawan elders (the healthier generation) eat an average of seven to ten servings of vegetables and fruit, seven servings of grain, and two servings of soy products each day—things like local bitter cucumbers, or *goya*, and sweet potatoes. The older group also eat fish several times a week and about one ounce of poultry or pork daily, and minimal dairy products.

So what knocked the Okinawa folks off of the pedestal? A major contributor to the decline in their position is the embracing of a more modern disregard for proven health habits, especially among 20 to 64-year-olds. The average life expectancy in all of Japan is 86.25 for women and 79.59 for men. Japan is one of the most rapidly aging societies in the world. Twenty-five percent of the population is age 65 or older. In the U.S., according to the CDC, life expectancy is 76.2 years for men and 80 years for women. Hawaii has the highest life expectancy in the U.S. at 78 for men and 84.7 for women.

Let's examine the "new" number one city for life expectancy. Nagano is a city of 2.15 million, almost the size of Connecticut, located in the Japanese Alps, an area which experiences long, harsh winters. Women in Nagano prefecture can expect to live an average of 87.2 years, while men can look forward to living 80.9 years. (Life expectancy in Connecticut is 2.3 years less for men and 4.3 years less for women.)

At first glance, Nagano would seem an unlikely setting for a long and healthy life. In the post-war era, men in particular suffered from high rates of stroke, heart attack, and cerebral aneurysm (rupturing vessels in the brain). Some analysts say that it was the high intake of salt in their diet, which primarily came from pickling their homegrown vegetables—they consumed three times the daily maximum of salt that we suggest in the US. Not surprising they had a high incidence of strokes. In fact, in 1981, they were the number one city to have a stroke in.

For Nagano, the first step in changing this whole scenario was a campaign to reduce salt consumption and promote a healthier diet and lifestyle. The government now conducts regular home visits to measure the salt content in daily meals and make dietary recommendations to citizens. This region of 2.1 million people now has some 4,500 volunteers who host seminars and clinics at supermarkets, shopping malls, and community centers. Public health officials in Japan have a motto of "improve your diet, stay active, and continue to work." Local leaders have developed a network of more than 100 walking routes to encourage people to stay active. Takuji Shirasawa, M.D., who teaches at the Department of Aging Control Medicine at Juntendo University in Tokyo, says, "The key is not just to live longer, but to stay healthy longer."[193]

Community and government efforts paid off rather rapidly. By 1990, life expectancy had risen to three years for men and three-and-a-half for women. Well done, Nagano!

Nagano's remarkable longevity is no doubt largely because of vigorous lifestyle encouragement by Japanese officials. Nagano has the highest number of people over 65 still working—nearly one in four people over 65 are still in the workforce the, highest rate in Japan. "We don't really know if people in Nagano continue to work because they are healthy, or if they are healthy because they continue to work," says Hiroko Akiyama, a professor at the University of Tokyo's Institute of Gerontology.

BOTTOM LINE: Eat the Okinawa diet, cut salt intake back, get into an aerobic exercise program, and have some meaningful activity in the later part of your life. Maybe even retire later than you planned!

---

[193] http://www.aarp.org/health/healthy-living/info-2014/longevity-secrets-from-japan.html

# RESISTANCE TRAINING

Although aerobic exercise has traditionally been emphasized for its health benefits, research increasingly suggests that associated resistance training also has favorable effects on coronary risk factors, cardiovascular health, and other physiological and psychosocial functions. The American Heart Association recommends the inclusion of resistance training for healthy persons of all ages, and for many patients with chronic diseases, including cardiovascular disease. Programs that include a single set of eight to ten different exercises performed two to three days a week have been shown to be beneficial. That is what you should shoot for. A greater frequency of training is an option, and additional gain is usually small.

A repetition range of eight to twelve is recommended for healthy participants younger than 50 to 60 years of age. To reduce the risk of injury, 10 to 15 repetitions at a lower relative resistance is generally recommended for cardiac patients and healthy participants over 50 to 60 years of age. Higher intensity efforts, meaning heavier weights, may increase the risk of musculoskeletal injury.

Designing a training plan? Here are the suggested steps to designing your resistance exercise-training program:

**Decide where you will lift.**

Working out at home is often the most time-efficient and practical solution. What equipment will you need? At home you will have to make some choices. Use solid dumbbells, since the plate-loading type can be a little dangerous. Solid hex dumbbells are more practical and may be less expensive. Round dumbbells tend to roll around and may pose a problem.

If you choose to work out at a gym, you'll find a wide variety of dumbbells and machines. Trainers are available and could be vey helpful to get you started.

**Define your goals.**

For most beginners, the goals are typically to tone up and get stronger. The good news is that any lifting will give you both, and you can expect strength gains in just a few weeks. Tone comes later, and how much muscle you see depends on how much excess body fat you have.

**Be consistent.**

We know that consistency is important in resistance training. Like any other activity involving the muscles of the body, a regular routine should be established. Older individuals who do resistance training quickly lose their muscle strength and endurance when there are periods of cessation of the exercise. Re-establishing the training effect is more difficult the older a person is. Younger people can take short breaks and catch up to their previous level of conditioning more quickly.

**Get help.**
The best help will come from a professional trainer, but that is usually not practical. Going on the Internet to various sources is a good thing to do. There are varied and many programs you can find there. Remember, the dictionary is the only place where success comes before work!

BOTTOM LINE: Resistance training will help range of motion, improve joint stability, cause toning, and provide strength that is lost as one ages.

# RESERVE

Nowadays we have to use all of our mentality, vitality, and functionality that we can muster. It is a different world we live in. And it ain't goin' to get any better. Oh, for the good old days, when we could coast. Although, if you want to go way back, the "good old days" were when you had to take your musket with you to protect yourself against the Indians when you went out in the woods to "meditate."

My grandparents could tell me about the good old days when, 107 years ago, only 14 percent of the homes in the U.S. had a bathtub. You had to wait in line to use the tub—the tub with the same water the other siblings had used. Most women only washed their hair once a month, and used Borax or egg yolks for shampoo. Only 8 percent of homes had a telephone. There were only 8,000 cars in the U.S., and only 144 miles of paved roads. More than 95 percent of all births in the U.S. took place at home. Ninety percent of all U.S. doctors had no college education. The top three leading causes of death were pneumonia, influenza, and tuberculosis . Stroke and heart disease followed infections on the list. Marijuana, heroin, and morphine were all available over the counter at the local corner drugstore. People didn't lock their doors. If your family had a few clothes to wear, a roof over their head, and three square meals a day, life was good!

For me, the good old days were when I routinely got my brothers hand-me-downs, and when I had my tonsils out on the kitchen table with my father administering the ether while the doctor did the surgery. Those were the days when parents could send their kids out to play and never see them again until supper. They were safe, except for occasionally falling and sustaining a cut or broken wrist. In 1907 there were about 230 reported murders in the entire U.S.

In my boyhood years, we had only one phone, and it was on a party line. Before you could dial, you had to listen and make sure a stranger wasn't already using the line. If it was not busy, the first thing you heard was, "Operator." She would then connect you to the person you wanted to talk to. The only thing that was delivered to our home was milk—no FedEx or Domino's Pizza. Life was good!

I would suggest that quality of life is about much more than simply what we have. It's about how satisfying we perceive our lifestyle to be. The real challenges come with extreme losses like divorce, death of loved ones, loss of a job, and loss of health and physical independence. Those situations have been with us and will continue to be with us forever. Aging, which we all do every day, can be one of life's toughest moments.

As we grow older, every tissue and every organ is involved in "planned death," or apoptosis, under the direction of nature. Some organs take a more significant hit than others. I guess you could say we rust, in a sense. Sensory changes include a decline in sight and peripheral vision, hearing, smell, and taste. The losses may be neither total nor rapid. The amount of muscle begins to decrease, beginning around age 30, and continues throughout life. More severe muscle loss, called sarcopenia, accelerates around late mid-life. Then, there are cognitive changes, which concern all of us.

Organs have a reserve ability to function beyond their usual needs. For example, the heart of a 20-year-old is capable of pumping about 10 times the amount of blood that is actually needed to keep the body alive. After age 30, an average of 1 percent of this reserve is lost each year.

With this as a background, I will now try to explain what I think is one of the most important sections of the book. The subject is *reserve*. Every organ has its own reserve.

In general terms, *reserve* is the ability to "bounce back" or to recover a previous level of function after an insult to a tissue or organ. Here is a theoretical example that closely approximates a study done about mobility and muscle reserve. Let's take 100 twenty-five year old people and put them in group A. Then let's take 100 seventy-year-old people and call them group B. By design, each person will have no impairment that would invalidate the experiment, except the reserve, which is being studied.

We will measure off a specific distance, say 50 yards. Groups A and B will walk as fast as they can, and each person's performance will be measured. Both groups will do their best, and after the walking they will be tested scientifically to see how much energy and performance is left. Group A will not have exhausted the performance of muscle and cardiopulmonary systems, although they tried. The older group, group B, will have little if any reserve left, through no fault of their own. Group A will be found to have 30 percent reserve left over. Group B, nothing left.

The loss of reserve, mobility, and strength marches on in all of us. Watch a three-year-old fall down. The child barely hits the floor before he is up again. Many elderly fall and can't get up, even if it means ultimate death.

As for the brain, it is at the mercy of other organs such as the heart for its supply of blood, the kidneys to keep metabolic balance, the lungs for oxygenation, etc.

I have seen older patients undergo surgery that would be routine for a robust 30 or 40 year old and become and remain confused for hours, if not days. Infections may challenge the remaining brain reserve of the older individual. So reserve is what you call on when handling physiologic stress and environmental changes. There are a myriad of environmental challenges the brain must respond to. An important point to make is that there are a number of medications that may be linked to causing cognitive impairment by inducing confusion, disorientation, memory loss, amnesia, and even coma.

An example of the impact on the brain from external environmental sources is made clearer by relating the example of the great composer Ludwig van Beethoven. An analysis of Beethoven's hair found lead concentration 100 times greater than normal. He may have been exposed to the lead in his drinking water and in water he swam in at spas. The lead poisoning could explain Beethoven's' erratic behavior in the years before his death in 1827, including his long, unkempt hair, filthy appearance, and fits of temper.

As we age, the ceiling begins to close in. Through well-directed choices you can prevent some untoward events, and slow others.

BOTTOM LINE: Environment, genetics, comorbid diseases, and lifestyles all influence reserve.

# THE FUTURE PHYSICIAN

As doctors, when we enter the room where the patient is seated, we may or may not shake hands or be forthcoming with a cheery greeting. Instead, we might be focused on the computer screen. The computer holds about everything we put into it and gives back what we desire, which includes things like vital signs, laboratory values, BMI, medications, last colonoscopy, information from the visit to the cardiologist, vaccination history, last eye exam, last Pap smear, which exercise program the patient is on (or has abandoned), which relative had what disease, and what color of toenail polish a woman likes to use.

That is all good, but the required list of these items grows larger and larger until the physician has the "guts of the exam" squeezed so tight there is little time to hear what the patient wants to communicate.

Today's reality is that electronic documentation takes precedence over the once meaningful interactive encounter between patient and doctor. The primary care provider is becoming a master at checking boxes, asking questions, and making accurate entries into the patient's electronic health record. I don't think patients know that their day with the doctor's computer not only may benefit them, but that their information is used to evaluate the provider's productivity and performance. Your "computer doctor" receives a report card on how he practices medicine. The computer gives him all kinds of information that can be analyzed for whatever purpose. He can do all these kinds of things on computers. Your doctor often gets bonuses (even from the government) on how well he can enter all of the bits of information into the computer. The tools we have measure provider performance as well as patient outcome.

I am not sure that we will ever get back to where we once were, and that may be for the better—or it could be for the worse. Our present medical knowledge and the way we treat patients is ever changing, and the "good folks" (our bosses) are trying to keep up with the change.

One man's opinion, whether it be mine or another physician trying to analyze and perhaps help formulate healthcare policy, does have value, but nonetheless, is just still one man's opinion. I found an article in the editorial section of JAMA by Jordan J. Cohen, MD, to be very thought provoking. "Will Changes in the MCAT and USMLE Ensure That Future Physicians Have What It Takes?" contains a great number of truths. It admits that we in the U.S. are not number one in healthcare, but it neglects to mention that we are ranked 26th in the world in life expectancy.

Dr. Cohen says, "It is now clear that the once-vaunted U.S. healthcare system was costing too much money, producing less than outstanding outcomes, failing to meet acceptable levels of quality and safety, and delivering substantially different standards of care depending on where someone lived, how much money they made, to what racial or what ethnic group they belonged, and whether they had health insurance."[194] In a word, we call that *rationing*. I see rationing becoming more of a challenge as time goes on, and with the government attempting to put the healthcare dollar in the most useful spot, rationing will be easily recognized as what it really is—offering care to some, refusing care to others.

He continues, "These challenges are unprecedented because newly minted physicians will not be working with a broken healthcare system requiring a few fixes, but rather with an outmoded legacy system that is inherently incapable of dealing effectively with the very problems it has produced. To lead, manage, and implement the transformative changes required, future physicians will need skills previous generations had scant use for."[195]

In thinking about the future, Dr. Cohen mentions a few things we need to think about in order to fix the problems with our medical system:

1. How to use resources parsimoniously
2. How to recognize and seize opportunities for improving the processes and end results of care
3. How to apply systems seeking to insure optimal patient outcomes, since computers are the cornerstones of the delivery of healthcare

Physicians will have to be less driven by business protocols and unnecessary technology, and more dedicated to compassionate service.

Dr. Cohen concludes. "A passionate devotion to serving others will be essential if 'tomorrows physicians' are to remain steadfast in adhering to those values despite the wrenching changes in the financing and organization in physicians services."[196]

What of "tomorrow's physicians?" What does the person who pursues a medical career face, and how will that impact you and me? Because of the tremendous debt a medical student will have when getting out and into practice, students with high debt seem less likely to pursue family practice and primary care specialties and instead will most likely seek specialties with higher incomes to pay back the financial commitments they have made. This is bad news, because the U.S. needs primary care physicians in addition to specialists.

Students from low-income/minority backgrounds and those with other financial responsibilities are discouraged from even applying to medical school because of the prohibitive cost and the resources it takes to get started on this career path. The Association of American Medical Colleges' Survey of Resident/Fellow Stipends and Benefits Report, 2013-2014, concludes that the average educational debt of indebted graduates of the class of 2013 will be $169,901. The report also tells us that the actual cost of repaying these loans will be much higher. For example, the repayment on a $175,000 loan could ultimately

---

[194] http://jama.jamanetwork.com/article.aspx?articleid=1787395

[195] http://jama.jamanetwork.com/article.aspx?articleid=1787395

[196] http://jama.jamanetwork.com/article.aspx?articleid=1787395

range from $326,000 to $492,000, depending on forbearance through residency and length of time taken to pay off the loan.[197]

In 2000, first-year out-of-state medical student tuition averaged $10,575, and in 2013, it was up to $63,090. When I was a sophomore in medical school I married a talented, wonderful young lady, Laura, and she was the big reason we graduated with no debt. She was the secretary to the head of the physics department, and as I graduated with my MD degree, she got her PHT (Putting Husband Through). Although, if my memory is accurate, my in-state medical student tuition for the University of Utah College of Medicine was under $500 per semester.

Our future physicians not only face a system that needs fixing, more information than they can assimilate, and the overburden of technology, but significant personal challenges we cannot possibly imagine.

BOTTOM LINE: For the caregiver and patient alike, there are no shortages of problems to overcome in our future.

---

[197] https://www.aamc.org/download/359792/data/2013stipendsurveyreportfinal.pdf

# AGING

The icon for longevity, Methuselah ("Man of the Spear") lived 969 years. He was the son of Enoch and fathered Lamech at the age of 187; Lamech fathered Noah at the age of 182, and thus it is calculated that Methuselah died in the year of the great flood. What was his secret for long life (and did he really live that long)?
Genesis 1:29:

*And God said, Behold, I have given you every herb bearing seed, which is upon the face of all the earth, and every tree, in the which is the fruit of a tree yielding seed; to you it shall be for meat.*

One could assume that Methuselah's diet was dramatically different than ours and every other Western society's. It appears it could have been a vegetarian diet. We will probably never know the answers to our questions, but the Bible shows that human lifespan diminishing radically after the Great Flood. After the Flood, consuming the flesh of animals became the norm, an acceptable way of life.

Recent advances in medical technology and scientific understanding have boosted average life expectancy to unprecedented levels. More than 34 million people in the United States are 65 years of age, and 4 million are over 85 years of age. The demographics have now classified the elderly into three groups:

- Those 65 to 75 years of age are "young-old."
- Those 75 to 85 years of age are now the "middle age" of the elderly.
- "Old-old" is reserved for the rapidly expanding group of those over 85 years of age.

In fact, those over 85 currently comprise the fastest growing segment of the population. This group's numbers are expected to double within the next 30 years. Aging may well begin before 65 years of age, though. The AARP accepts membership as early as 50 years old. Thus, growing old can be a lifelong process. It is not a destination but a pathway.

Down the road a piece—but sooner than most appreciate—the major health problems of the United States will be directly related to the process of senescence, where the aging process itself, along with accumulation of disease, will constitute a major burden of illness. The word *senescence* is derived from the Latin word *senescere*, meaning "to grow old." The changes that occur as we grow old are due to the accumulative molecular and cellular breakdown products (free radicals) which disrupt metabolism over a period of time, resulting in deterioration and eventually death.

We are all older today than we were yesterday—not particularly a brilliant statement, nonetheless, an eye opener for those who think they are immortal. And there are some in our midst who believe it! Young folks, for example.

If you're into the science of this, let's look at three major cause of aging: oxidative stress, glycation, and an overactive sympathetic nervous system.

### Oxidative Stress

Oxidative stress is caused by an imbalance of oxygen in metabolism and the toxic byproducts of that reaction, primarily in the form of released free radicals. Free radicals damage the DNA of proteins and lipids. These oxidants are produced normally when we breathe, and also result from inflammation, infection, and consumption of alcohol and cigarettes, as well as physical inactivity. Take a look at an apple after it has been sliced and exposed to the air. It becomes brown as a consequence of rapid aging—or oxidation.

### Glycation

Another factor in aging is glycation. This happens when the glucose (sugar) from what we eat binds to some of our DNA, proteins, and lipids, leaving them impotent to perform their genetically directed functions.

### Overactive Sympathetic Nervous System

The sympathetic nervous system's "flight or fight" mechanisms are of course necessary, but also cause the body wear and tear.

However, look far enough and you can always find good news. The good news in this case is that human beings have a superior DNA reparative mechanism compared to other living animals—the presence of antioxidants, for example, is one of the blessings of an efficient body (see the chapter on antioxidants).

James L. Kirkland, M.D., Ph.D. at the Mayo Clinic states, "We view aging as a major driver of illness and healthcare costs. We're asking if we can reduce the period of illness toward the end of life."[198] This period of life Dr. Kirkland speaks of should be of interest to all of us. It has a name: "compression of morbidity."

When it's our time to "go," we all hope it happens overnight, in our sleep, at a very old age. Not only do we want to "go" rapidly and painlessly, we would want to be functional, productive, and happy up to that night we retire to our bed. Unfortunately, 80 to 90 percent of deaths come from chronic causes, most of which start a number of years before that last final heartbeat.

Compression of morbidity means having as little illness, loss of function, and "bad hair days" as possible from the time significant decline in function and

---

[198] http://www.mayo.edu/research/discoverys-edge/uncovering-clues-about-aging-process

quality of life begins until death. The time frame within which this happens for the average American is up to 10 years. Making this change from good health to death appropriate and meaningful is called "successful aging." The glass-half-full folks" call it "successful dying."

Normal aging is marked by a decline of motor function and mobility and by the impairment of specific cognitive functions. In fact, much of normal aging closely mimics the effects of immobilization and inactivity.

It doesn't take great intellect to figure out that the possibility of death has been holding pretty steady at 100 percent for some time. Roughly 100,000 people worldwide die each day of age-related causes. Death happens to all of us.

The longest documented human lifespan was of one Jeanne Calment of France, who lived from 1875 to 1997, putting her at 122 years, 164 days at the time of her death. Although she just passed away in recent decades, she was around long enough that in her youth, she is rumored to have met Vincent van Gogh.[199]

The ancient Greek poet Homer called old age "loathsome." In Greek mythology, the Greek God Tithonus lived forever, but when loathsome old age, with its full weight, fell upon him, and he experienced the ravages of aging, he could not move nor lift his limbs. He was put into what we now call "assisted living," and there he babbled endlessly and continued to remain in a continuous state of dependency.

Sometimes minimal, sometimes gigantic things occur as we age. The rate at which we age is very significant and takes us down that muddy road or that rosy path to the final day when our birth certificate expires. Aging often takes us right into retirement. One of the top desires, if not the top wishes, for the older individual is to be independent. Much of what we do during our productive working years is to plan, prepare, and remain independent. It is estimated that 43.5 million individuals in the United States provide in-home, long-term care for older adult family members with a chronic disease. The aging process effects many, even before we have been labeled "elderly."[200]

Otto von Bismarck, German Chancellor, established the arbitrary designation of retirement at 65 years of age in late 19th century Germany. Bismark knew that the program would cost little, because the average German worker never reached 65, and many of those who did lived only a few years beyond that age. Therefore, the social welfare program he proposed for retirees was of minimal cost to the public.

When the United States finally passed a social security law in 1935, the average life expectancy in America was only 61.7 years. In 1900, there were 3.1 million in the U.S. 65 or older. The 65-and-older population jumped 15.1 percent between 2000 and 2010, compared with a 9.7 percent increase for the total U.S. population. People age 65 and older now make up 13 percent of the total population,

---

[199] http://en.wikipedia.org/wiki/Oldest_people

[200] http://jama.jamanetwork.com/issue.aspx?journalid=67&issueid=929845

compared with 12.4 percent in 2000 and 4.1 percent in 1900.[201] This is my personal prayer: "May He keep those young folks working to pay Medicare bills, and fund my monthly social security checks."

An aging population does have a considerable social impact. We are very aware of the present-day financial implications of an aging America. The loss of the older group as tax revenue and the increased pressure on the younger working class is going to cause government to make some pretty tough choices. Needless to say, we who are over 65 will be the ones left on our own, relatively speaking. More reason to depend on yourself! Stay with me, as I am building a case that will help you see the need to be more involved in your future.

Earlier, I mentioned successfully aging. If you are depending upon your parent's good health and genes to help you live the highest form of a healthy life, be careful. Environment and lifestyle are far more important than genes in regard to aging. As you will read over and over again, environment and lifestyle are modifiable, and the opportunities for change in these areas are abundant. Even with a strong genetic predisposition toward a particular risk factor or disease such as colon cancer or heart attacks, each of us can modify our genetic susceptibility. In general, genetic forces on health decline with advancing age, while the influence of environmental factors increases.

Successful aging is more than having a short time of ill health before death. The concept of successful aging was popularized in the 1980s. To agree on the way we measure successful aging is problematic. One could reasonably think about successful aging as being able to appropriately adapt to, and reshape, life's events through mind, body, and spiritual methods. Others in the medical field will emphasize plasticity and variation in making life both comfortable and productive.

I favor the idea of successful aging as consisting of four components: low probability of disease or disability, high cognitive and physical function capacity, optimal reserve, and active engagement with life. That is the way I see myself fitting on the continuum of aging.

These four elements will insure the most desired part of our later years: independence. As we position ourselves to attain the independent life, the "good life" will become a reality. Rowe and Kahn, oft quoted experts on aging and the elderly, note that, "When older people are asked about their hopes, aspirations, and goals for their senior years, they simply note that they want to remain independent and continue to take care of themselves."[202] Then Rowe and Kahn ask the question, "Should one expect to lose one's faculties and become dependent on others; in effect, to age normally?" That is not my idea of normal aging. Even today, I'm working on being independent! Tomorrow, I'm doing the same thing. I'm going down to the city recreation center to do my 500-calorie "burn" on the stationary bike.

---

201 http://money.usnews.com/money/retirement/articles/2012/01/09/65-and-older-population-soars
202 http://www.instituteoflifestylemedicine.org/file/doc/publications/articles_by/NormalAging_Phillips.pdf

Physiologically, we begin to decline at 30 years of age, or thereabouts. Physiologic decline is around 1.5 percent per year, depending on the organ. But age also brings anatomic changes. Brain weight and blood flow to the brain eventually decrease by 20 percent. The number of fibers and nerves decrease by 37 percent, and brain volume shrinks up to 1 percent every year after age 65.

Building cognitive reserve delays the onset of memory loss, and research suggests that novel and complex brain activities can delay cognitive decline and extend lifespan.

Poor education, poor social interaction, and lives devoid of mental simulation result in less cognitive reserve. Remember, we call on our reserve at various points in our lives when we experience stress, emotional trauma, physical injury, and insomnia, to mention just a few.

The linear decline in organ reserve takes the individual to a point at which function must be inadequate to support life—that point apparently being when organ reserve is reduced to approximately 20 percent above the function required for the maintenance of basic life processes.

In *Primary Psychiatry*: Edward Phillips MD and Donald A Davidoff, PhD report that "In reality, only a fraction of the normal decline in physical functioning is directly related to chronological aging. Control subjects in their seventh decade studied over 10 years were found to have maximal oxygen consumption declines of 12 percent over the less active. On the other hand, age-matched runners showed declines of only 5.5 percent."[203] Oxygen consumption is one way that body efficiency can be measured. The higher the level, the "healthier" the system. Runners have half the decline in cardiovascular efficiency than sedentary folks have.

What about the brain? Dr. Vincent Fortanasce, world-renowned neurologist, psychiatrist, and rehabilitation specialist, states, "Mental agility begins declining around age 24. But there is a big difference between agility and capacity. I may be slower, but what I know now far outweighs what I knew at 24."[204] "Fortanasce also says, "Some individuals perform their greatest creative work late in life. Verdi, for example, composed Othello at 73 and Falstaff at 79."[205] Though we often use our age as an excuse, it is not always a very good one.

Physiologic age is more important than calendar age. We can look into a number of metrics and get some idea of our physiologic age. Body fat, either too much or too, little gives us an idea of our physiological age. Muscle mass and strength is another measurement.

Aerobic fitness is one of the better measurements of health and predicted mortality. A good aerobic fitness test is the six-minute walk test. If you cannot walk beyond 332 meters or 360 yards in less than six minutes, you have an increased mortality rate. This is a good predictor of moderately severe poor

[203] http://www.instituteoflifestylemedicine.org/file/doc/publications/articles_by/NormalAging_Phillips.pdf
[204] http://www.amednews.com/article/20081117/health/311179980/4/
[205] http://www.brainhq.com/news/physical-and-mental-exercise-help-keep-brain-fit

physical conditioning.

Measurable changes in cognitive efficiency do not appear until after 50 years of age. It is estimated that overall intelligence does not significantly decline until the seventh decade of life. In order to combat cognitive decline, you must constantly challenge yourself. "When you challenge the brain with new skills and new ways of doing things, it increases connections in the brain," says Ericka P. Simpson, MD, a neurologist and director of ALS clinical research division at the Methodist Hospital System.[206]

Dr. Fortanasce tells us "Exercise can actually increase neurogenesis (new brain cell growth) and increase the size of the hippocampus (part of the memory mechanism)." In his clinic, he promotes isometrics and weight-bearing exercise. In a 2006 study in the *Journal of Aging and Physical Activity*, Brandeis University researchers found that strength training increased participants' working memory spans.[207] The higher the level of resistance, the more memory improved, suggesting that strength training benefits not only the muscles but also the mind.

*Nature Neuroscience* published research by University College London scientists in 2013 proving that complex brain processes that enable memorization and replication of activities (like playing an instrument or learning to ride a bike) require complicated sequences of movements involving many muscles. Pianists in the study who learned and practiced from an early age were proven less likely to later be diagnosed with cognitive neurodegenerative changes.[208] My own mother made quite sure all of her kids took piano lessons, although only my sister Cathy retained this skill. Perhaps this is why she is so mentally sharp to this day.

Christian D. Larson was an American New Thought leader and teacher as well as a prolific author of metaphysical and New Thought books. Here's a quote by him:

*Promise yourself to be so strong that nothing can disturb your peace of mind. Look at the sunny side of everything and and make your optimism come true. Think only of the best, work only for the best. Forget the mistakes of the past and press on the greater achievements of the future. Give so much time to the improvement of yourself that you have no time to criticize others. Live in the faith that the whole world is on your side as long as you are true to the best that is in you.[209]*

Kermit Long relates a story about two men who were walking along a crowded sidewalk in a downtown business area. Suddenly one exclaimed; "Listen to the lovely sound of that cricket." But the other one could not hear. He

[206] http://www.amednews.com/article/20081117/health/311179980/4/

[207] http://www.amednews.com/article/20081117/health/311179980/4/

[208] http://www.amednews.com/article/20081117/health/311179980/4/

[209] http://christianlarson.wwwhubs.com

asked his companion how he could detect the sound of a cricket amid the din of the people and the traffic. The first man, who was a zoologist, had trained himself to listen to the voices of nature. But instead of explaining, he took a coin out of this pocket and dropped it on the sidewalk. A dozen people immediately began looking around. "We hear what we listen for."

In order to attain a full portion of happiness, we must listen and find the things in life that have meaning, even if it is the sound of a cricket.

I can't remember names as well as I used to, and I can't run or even walk as fast as I used to. Certainly, my joints are a little stiffer. I know that I cannot stay young, but I can always stay "fresh." For every measured loss there is an immeasurable gain. The success of old age depends upon what you are looking for and what your now thoroughly processed goals are.

Nouwen said:

*Pouring little bits of water on our dry land does not help, but that we find a living well if we reach deep enough beneath the surface of our own complaints. Are you willing to stoop down and consider the needs and desires of little children, to remember the weakness and loneliness of people who are going to stop asking how much your friends love you, and to ask yourself whether you love them enough, to bear in mind the things that other people have to bear in their hearts to trim your lamp so that it will give more light and less smoke, and to carry it in front of you so that your shadow will fall behind you, to make a grave for your ugly thoughts and a garden for your kind feelings, with the gate open?*[210]

If growing old catches you by surprise, don't blame God. He gave you plenty of warning. He also gave you plenty of advice!

BOTTOM LINE: You can't turn back the clock. But you can wind it up again. Nobody grows old by merely living a number of years. People grow old only by deserting their ideals. Years may wrinkle the skin, but to give up interest in life wrinkles the soul.

---

[210] *The Three Movements of the Spiritual Life: Reaching Out* , Henri J. M. Nouwen, Doubleday, New York, pp. 165

# ALZHEIMER'S DISEASE

So far, I've used a great deal of ink discussing morbidity and early death caused by obesity and overweight issues, bad food selection, and a sedentary lifestyle. You have read a great deal about the decline of cognitive ability and what causes this phenomenon. It is altogether fitting that we now discuss Alzheimer's disease, one of the causes of dementia.

I once heard a saying: "Memory is responsible for the past, plans for the future, and appreciates and makes the present work."

Everyone wants a good memory, so the subject of Alzheimer's disease and dementia should get your attention. Before launching too deeply into the subject, let's come to an understanding of the words *dementia* and *Alzheimer's disease*.

Dementia is a general disease category—much like fruit is a category—which contains a number of different items. Generally speaking, dementia refers to a decline in memory or other thinking skills (cognition) severe enough to reduce a person's ability to perform everyday activities. Depending on whom you ask, Alzheimer's disease (AD) causes 60 to 80 percent of dementia cases. Alzheimer's disease is the apple, if you will. Other causes of dementia include Lewy body dementia (the pear), vascular dementia (the orange), frontotemporal dementia (the peach), etc. Most dementias have very similar clinical manifestations, but there are different signs and symptoms that tend to separate one from the other.

Five percent of those 65 and older have dementia, while there is a 40 percent chance of having dementia at age 85 and older. Let us direct our attention to the nation's sixth leading cause of death, Alzheimer's disease.

From the Alzheimer's Association, we get the following statistics:
1. Alzheimer's disease is the sixth leading cause of death in the United States.
2. More than 5 million Americans are living with Alzheimer's disease.
3. One in three seniors dies with Alzheimer's or another dementia.
4. In 2012, 15.4 million caregivers provided more than 17.5 billion hours of unpaid care.
5. In 2013, Alzheimer's cost the U.S. $203 billion annually, with expectations that in 2050 that figure will be $1.2 trillion.
6. More than 60 percent of Alzheimer's and dementia caregivers rate the emotional stress of caregiving as high or very high; more than one-third of caregivers report symptoms of depression.[211]

---

[211] http://www.alz.org/downloads/facts_figures_2013.pdf

For another viewpoint that may give us more hope and encouragement, the *New York Times* reported on a study performed in England and Wales that found that dementia rates among people over the age of 65 in those two countries has plummeted by 25 percent over the past two decade, "a trend that researchers say is probably occurring across developed countries and that could have major social and economic implications for families and societies."[212]

Very early in life we begin to lose some of our cerebral capabilities. This cognitive vitality, as we will call it, is what we all hope to maintain, if not magnify. Around age 20 we begin to see the loss of cognitive vitality in four areas: word recall, matrix reasoning, spatial relations, and pattern comprehension. From 20 to 70, there is a 70 percent decline in these areas of cognition. Fortunately, the loss is offset by our gains in wisdom and experience.

How might we prevent cognitive decline with aging? I will not discuss all of the ramifications of prevention and treatment of Alzheimer's disease, but only a few I think are important. I would like to introduce you to Dr. Gary Small, director of the UCLA Longevity Center at the university's Semel Institute for Neuroscience & Human Behavior. He was named one of the world's leading innovators in science and technology, and is a professor of psychiatry at UCLA's David Geffen School of Medicine. His book *The Alzheimer's Prevention Program* is certainly worth purchasing.

Dr. Small says, "If everyone in the U.S. adopted just one additional healthy lifestyle habit (perhaps took a brisk walk every other day or ate fish twice a week), within five years we could anticipate one million fewer cases of Alzheimer's disease than otherwise expected."[213]

I like that "brisk walk" idea. Another study looked at a group of people who walked for six months and found them to have cognitive function improvements and an increase in brain size by appropriate brain imaging.

Dr. Small also said, "A recent study indicated that physical exercise several times a week over a two-year period lowered a person's future risk for memory decline by 46 percent. Eating antioxidant fruits and vegetables such as blueberries and broccoli for a four-year period reduced dementia by 44 percent. People who spend time doing complex mental tasks during midlife decreased their dementia risk by as much as 48 percent."[214]

Much more can be said about lifestyle changes and the areas Dr. Small addresses. Social engagement, for instance, not only improves cognition more quickly, but may also delay the onset of dementia. Social engagement means getting out and associating in various forms with other people in other situations. It is the antithesis of the "stay at home" paradigm.

We have evidence to suggest that social activity and a supportive network

---

[212] http://www.nytimes.com/2013/07/17/health/study-finds-dip-in-dementia-rates.html?_r=1&

[213] *The Alzheimer's Prevention Program: Keep Your Brain Healthy for the Rest of Your Life,* Gary Small, Workman Publishing Company; Upd Rep edition (December 11, 2012)

[214] *The Alzheimer's Prevention Program: Keep Your Brain Healthy for the Rest of Your Life,* Gary Small, Workman Publishing Company; Upd Rep edition (December 11, 2012)

results in better cognitive function. The higher the level of social engagement in the older person, the better the cognitive function. As one gets older, it is common to withdraw from social contacts and situations that a person once sought and was comfortable with. There are many reasons for this, including loss of confidence in a social setting, depression, and cognitive decline.

The Women's Health Initiative Memory Study, supported by the National Heart, Lung and Blood Institute, looked at omega-3 fatty acids levels in the red blood cells of 1,111 women an average of 78 years old. (Omega-3 fatty acids, remember, are found in fish such as tuna, salmon, mackerel, and sardines.) MRI brain scans were done to measure the participants' brain volumes eight years after the study began. Older women with the highest levels of omega-3 fatty acids had better anatomical preservation of their brains as they aged than those with the lowest levels. The suggestion, according to the study, is that higher omega-3 fatty acid blood levels may lessen cognitive decline. By the way, that comes from food, not supplements.

Brain reserve is the ability to tolerate the age-related changes and other disease processes without developing clear clinical signs or symptoms. Increasing this reserve is influenced by the level of education, complexity of work, extent of social network, level of engagement, and amount of leisure activities. We are realizing more and more that leisure activities—physical, mental, and social—are important in our lives for many reasons.

There is a great deal of controversy and misinformation, and a vast expanse of confusion, about foods and supplements. Even most experts agree that supplements are probably a waste of money when it comes to their cognitive value. We do know that dietary habits need to be established years ahead of the potential onset of Alzheimer's disease. So, get after it and change your eating habits now. Now is none too soon!

BOTTOM LINE: Begin early on in your efforts to prevent dementia. Eat a well-rounded diet rich in fruits and vegetables, keep mentally challenged, and develop or keep up a strong exercise program.

# ALCOHOL

There is an idea circulating about that alcohol will reduce the risks associated with heart disease. In fact, there are some in the medical field who suggest that alcohol, particularly red wine, is heart-healthy. The theory that the antioxidants in red wine increase levels of high-density lipoprotein (HDL) cholesterol ("good" cholesterol), which protects the endothelium (lining) of vessels. Additionally, alcohol is thought to reduce low-density lipoprotein (LDL) cholesterol ("bad" cholesterol) and possibly prevent blood clots.

How much alcohol must one drink to get these suggested benefits? The amount of alcohol associated with beneficial effects ranges from one to two and a half drinks a day, according to the research.

I've heard many people speak and have read many dissertations about alcohol's cardiovascular benefits, and I've noticed that experts always add the caveat: "Be careful about encouraging anyone to start drinking for the cardiovascular benefits if they presently don't drink."

Now let's hear the other side of the alcohol story. Reducing alcohol consumption in the United States is an important and underemphasized cancer prevention strategy. The Public Health Institute tells us that "When viewed in the broad context, alcohol results in 10 times as many deaths as it prevents in the United States even after one considers possible beneficial effects of low-level use for cardiovascular disease and diabetes."[215] I think this view, along with the voices of many others, puts to rest the idea that one should consume alcohol— even small amounts.

A U.S. Department of Health and Human Services brochure called "Rethinking Drinking" tells us that "Alcohol plays a part in about 60 percent of fatal burn injuries, drownings, and homicides; 50 percent of severe trauma injuries and sexual assaults; and 40 percent of fatal motor vehicle crashes, suicides, and fatal falls."[216]

The health problem list is long: blood clotting problems, an increased workload of the heart associated with cirrhosis of the liver, liver disease, atrial fibrillation, myocarditis, cardiomyopathy, high blood pressure, strokes, central nervous system degeneration, several types of cancer, and so forth. Drinking during pregnancy can cause brain damage and other serious problems in the baby. The combined use of tobacco, cigarettes, and alcohol appears to increase the risk of many of these clinical abnormalities.

Jürgen Rehm, PhD, WCR at The Centre for Addictions and Mental Health in Toronto, Ontario, Canada declared, "We have known for a long time that

---

[215] http://www.phi.org/news-events/411/drinking-causes-35-of-cancer-deaths-more-than-from-melanoma-new-study-finds

[216] http://pubs.niaaa.nih.gov/publications/RethinkingDrinking/Rethinking_Drinking.pdf

alcohol causes esophageal cancer, but the relationship with other tumors, such as breast cancer, has come to our attention only in the past 10 to 15 years."[217]

The more alcohol a person drinks, the higher the risk. In an article in *Medscape Oncology*, Laura A. Stokowski, RN, MS discusses a meta-analysis of 222 studies totaling 92,000 light drinkers and 60,000 nondrinkers with cancer, which showed that light drinking was associated with higher risk for mouth and throat cancer, esophageal carcinoma, and female breast cancer. From this meta-analysis, it was estimated that in 2004, worldwide, 5,000 deaths from mouth and throat cancer, 24,000 from esophageal carcinoma, and 5,000 from breast cancer were associated with light drinking.[218]

The American Journal of Public Health reported a study done in 2009 by David Nelson, MD, MPH, from the National Cancer Institute in Bethesda, Maryland showing that alcohol use accounted for approximately 3.5 percent of all cancer deaths in the United States, causing about 19,500 cancer deaths, with each alcohol-attributable death resulting in about 18 years of potential life lost.[219]

They also found that the more alcohol consumed, the greater the risk for related cancer death. "In sum, there is no apparent threshold when it comes to alcohol and cancer risk,"[220] the authors note. The majority of alcohol-attributable cancer deaths in women were from breast cancer, in men from upper airway and esophageal cancers.

Reducing alcohol consumption is "an important and underemphasized cancer prevention strategy,"[221] writes Dr. Nelson and colleagues. To underline this observation, a recent study cited alcohol as the eighth most common cause of cancer in the United States after smoking (33 percent of all cancers); overweight/obesity (20 percent); and diet, lack of exercise, occupation, viruses, and family history (5 percent each). Enough about alcohol.

BOTTOM LINE: The answer to the question "Is alcohol in any amount harmful?" is clearly yes. Seems prudent to avoid imbibing alcohol.

---

217

http://www.camh.ca/en/hospital/about_camh/influencing_public_policy/public_policy_submissions/alcohol/Documents/Alcohol%20Cancer%20Best%20Advice%20final.pdf

[218] http://www.medscape.com/viewarticle/824237_5

[219] http://www.ncbi.nlm.nih.gov/pmc/articles/PMC3673233/

[220] http://www.phi.org/news-events/411/drinking-causes-35-of-cancer-deaths-more-than-from-melanoma-new-study-finds

[221] http://ajph.aphapublications.org/doi/abs/10.2105/AJPH.2012.301199

# SMOKING

As far as I know, tobacco came on the scene in the U.S. when Columbus and his crew brought seeds and leaves back from their first journey to the Americas. Sir Walter Raleigh, born in about 1554, an English aristocrat, writer, poet, soldier, politician, and explorer, is well known for popularizing tobacco in England.

Tobacco has taken some big steps. First it was a curiosity, then an amusement, then it became an addiction, and now it's a big profitable business. More than 293 billion cigarettes were purchased in the United States in 2011. The idea of small farmers growing tobacco as their livelihood changed long ago. The number of tobacco-growing farms declined from more than 500,000 in the 1950s to about 10,000 in 2007. In 2011, including both cigarette and smokeless tobacco marketing, tobacco companies spent more than $24 million each day on advertising. If you think that number is big, think about our national debt. It is trillions (12 zeroes) of dollars. All I know is that both a billion and a trillion are way over a thousand!

Cigarettes known by the name of "100's" are typically three and three-quarter to four inches in length. To make it easier to calculate how long 293 billion cigarettes placed end-to-end would extend, lets say each one is four inches long. The earth's circumference at the equator—the widest point— is 24,901.55 miles. The number of cigarettes sold in the U.S. in the year 2011 would go around the earth about 742 times.

Throughout history, not everyone supported the cause of tobacco. King James I of England described smoking as "loathsome." The Qing Dynasty of China pronounced the death penalty upon those who smoked. At one time, Turkey also imposed a death penalty for smoking tobacco.

Smoking is certainly a lifestyle that carries with it much disease and misery. To list all of the problems it creates would be a major task, but to get a flavor of the lethality, you should know that cigarette smoking causes an estimated 400,000 deaths per year in the U.S. This figure is equivalent to two Boeing 2-class layout jets crashing each day. Worldwide smoking-related diseases kill around 6 million people each year. I remember the anthrax scare of 2001, which killed five people and infected 17 others, and how much of a problem that was for we Americans. Yet we live with the comparative equivalent of two jumbo jets crashing every day without doing anything about it.

The four leading causes of death—heart disease, cancer (particularly lung cancer), cerebrovascular disease, and chronic obstructive pulmonary disease (COPD)—are all strongly related to smoking. In general, the relative risk of death due to coronary heart disease in smokers is two to four times greater than that in persons who have never smoked. The yearly cost to the employer of one who smokes is about $3,800. This is primarily due to lost time at work. This is an often-unappreciated "fallout" from smoking.

And what about smoking's effects on others? *Secondhand smoke* is really a misnomer. It should be something like "ambient air tobacco inhalation," although, admittedly, that is a little bulky.

The CDC reports that since 1964, 2.5 million nonsmokers have died from exposure to secondhand smoke. In children 18 months and younger, sudden infant death syndrome (SIDS) is increased when adults in the home smoke. I don't know about you, but that certainly pulls at my heartstrings. An estimated 150,000 to 300,000 new cases of bronchitis and pneumonia occur annually as a result of secondhand smoking, in addition to about 7,500 to 15,000 hospitalizations.

In adults who have never smoked, secondhand smoke can cause cardiovascular disease and lung cancer. Nonsmokers who are exposed to secondhand smoke increase their lung cancer risk by 20 to 30 percent, and their heart disease risk by 25 to 30 percent.

It gets very personal when we know that secondhand smoke exposure caused nearly 34,000 heart disease deaths annually among adult nonsmokers in the period of 2005 to 2009.[222] I have had a few of those types of patients in my years of practice.

I went to medical school from the years 1954 to 1958. That was a long time ago. Whenever I reference those days, I always tell my conversation partner that I put myself through medical school for the first two years by selling kerosene lamps. I vividly remember our histology teacher, during my second year of medical school, saying that the idea that smoking causes lung cancer was "bunk." Of course, he smoked. He added, "Dying of lung cancer correlates better with the number of telephones installed yearly." I don't know about the telephone poles, but I do know that smoking is the scourge of society.

Science has come a long way since then. You can maybe appreciate how difficult it was for science, politicians, and the pubic at large (influenced by the tobacco lords) to put tobacco in its place as the number one killer in terms of preventable diseases. It took us a while to catch on about smoking, and even longer to realize the effects on those of us who don't "firsthand smoke."

When it comes to smoking tobacco, it makes no difference whether your cancer stick of choice is a cigar or cigarette: there's no such thing as a safe degree of exposure. Remember, the lesser-of-two evils argument won't mean much when it's too late.

Some estimates say that tobacco products contain up to 4,000 chemicals coming from the burning of the product, some say it's additives inserted by the company, but most agree that it's the cigarette's "natural ingredients." All cigarettes contain carcinogens (cancer-producing elements).

Studies have shown that when people stop smoking, their risk of tobacco-related morbidity and mortality decreases significantly. If you stop smoking at age

---

[222] http://www.cdc.gov/tobacco/data_statistics/fact_sheets/secondhand_smoke/general_facts/

40, you will add 10 years to your life. If you stop smoking at age 50, you will add 5 years to your life.. And if you stop smoking at age 60, you will add 3 years to your life.

More than 180 million lives could be saved in just the first half of this century if the prevalence of current tobacco users were cut in half by 2020. That is a staggering figure! Rumor has it—and it may just be rumor—that for every minute you smoke, you cut off one minute of life. No other intervention for cardiovascular disease is likely to be as cost-effective as smoking cessation.

Tobacco tax is the second most effective way to cut down on smoking, but the number one motivator to stop smoking is to have a heart attack. We are told that after a heart attack that 60 to 70 percent of victims stop smoking. The sad commentary is that in one month, 27 percent are back smoking, and at the end of one year, if they are still alive, 48 percent return to smoking. Next is the roll of the physician in queering the patient: "Are you ready to stop smoking"—or similar questions. There are a number of methods that one might employ in trying to stop smoking. They include, but are by no means limited to, inhalants containing nicotine, nasal sprays, gum, and medications such as Zyban and Chantix. Support groups and formal governmental help is available.

There is much, much more that can be said about tobacco, but I will leave the subject for you to research so you can do what it takes to stop your use of tobacco.

BOTTOM LINE: If you are a smoker, seek appropriate help. If you have already quit, I probably should take you out to dinner! There is no risk-free level of secondhand smoke exposure; even brief exposure can be harmful to health.

# STRESS

Someone who is a "hot reactor" may have 20 to 30 stress episodes a day. One study indicated that psychological distress (stress) may lead to a 54 percent increase risk of cardiovascular disease over seven years. Anger and hostility cause even worse problems, with the risk of a heart attack increasing 230 percent in a 2-hour period following an episode of anger.[223] Stress reducers include but are not limited to humor, midday naps (bringing in a 37 percent reduction in stress), and exercise. Sounds to me like some fairly attractive therapeutic options.

The stress response is adaptive, born within us in a programmed cascade of physiological, immune, metabolic, sensory, and musculoskeletal actions that are triggered by real or perceived threats to our safety and health.

- Stress causes cortisone release, and higher doses of cortisone are injurious to vessels.
  Catecholamines, likewise, are released with excess stress. Catecholamines increase blood pressure and heart rate and cause one to be more vigilant and alert.
  Cytokines increase clotting within the vessels.
- And other chemicals used in reparative processes are secreted or released with pathological amounts of stress.

The repeated release and interactions of the above chemicals put a load on human homeostasis, and as a result, we most often end up with a "wear and tear" scenario. Over time, the accrued load contributes to the risk for adverse health consequences medicated by the stress chemicals, including excessive inflammation, which causes arterial lining damage predisposing us to heart attacks, strokes, etc.

Too much stress also lowers our immune response. Stress is reduced by knowing your purpose and having a life plan consistent with your values. Liking oneself has wide application in life. Successful aging has to do with balance and adjusting to life's challenges. To be known, to love, to love someone else blunts the adverse affects of stress. To feel like we are contributing to others and being in unison with other people is stress reducing.

In a study of 5,731 adult older men and women, researchers found that with a better-quality diet, the risk of depression was lessened, whereas a higher intake of processed and unhealthy foods was associated with increased anxiety.[224] Better-quality diets, incidentally, are easily found in this book. You'll

---

[223] Journal of Circulation 1995

[224] http://www.medscape.com/viewarticle/819974

noticed I haven't suggested any pills at this point in our story.

Recent research by a team of investigators, including researchers from University College of London in the United Kingdom, analyzed the data of 10,308 civil servants in the UK. Researchers in the Whitehall Study followed up with all of the subjects for 20 years, and health assessments were carried out over two to three year intervals. The researchers found that participants who showed depressive symptoms in the first one or two assessments demonstrated no increase risk of coronary heart disease. Indicating the long-term effects, those who had symptoms of depression in the third or fourth assessments showed a 100 percent increase in risk of coronary heart disease.[225]

Food for thought: Could your diet play a part in your mood disorder? "In a study of 5,731 adult and older men and women, the research team found a lower risk for depression among participants with better-quality diets, and increased anxiety was observed with a higher intake of processed and unhealthy foods."[226]

On a daily basis, you may feel like you are the only fire hydrant at the Westminster Dog Show. If so, try a new approach. For the incessant, chronic worrier, may I suggest you set aside five minutes daily just to worry, then walk away and forget the things you can't do anything about.

I also advise a trial of the mini-deep-breathing technique developed by Dr. Herbert Benson, interventional cardiologist and founder of The Mind-Body Institute at Harvard. Within one minute, this technique of deep breathing increases the calming parasympathetics, decreases heart rate, drops blood pressure, and declines cortisol.

Here's how to do it:
1. Take a deep breath, expanding it into the abdomen.
2. Hold it for the count of four.
3. Breathe out slowly.
4. Repeat and continue for one minute.

Doing this simple technique when you start to feel stressed will aid you in overcoming the frequent stress events we all encounter daily.

You can become good at it by creating a routine of setting aside a time and place for the breathing exercise every day. Choose a special place that is quiet, comfortable, and conducive to concentration. To find the relaxation response, shift your focus from your stresses to deeper, more pleasant thoughts. Make it a habit to practice this process for five to ten minutes a day.

BOTTOM LINE: Looking at life's balance is a good way to go. Playing and having fun are good balancing activities. Have clarity about who you are and what you want to accomplish in life.

---

[225] http://www.ucl.ac.uk/whitehalllll/history

[226] http://www.medscape.com/viewarticle/819974

# SLEEP

Stay awake! This could be the most important section of this book, because it has such a broad application. If you need to get a drink of water, get up and walk around, or maybe chew on a cracker in order to be alert, do it— anything to be able to devote your consciousness to that which you are now about to read.

In the New Testament (Acts 20:6-12), Paul traveled to Troas, and on the first day of the week, he preached unto them, "and continued his speech until midnight." A man called Eutychus fell into a deep sleep. We are not told whether he had narcolepsy, suffered from sleep deprivation, or was simply bored, but nonetheless, he was unable to keep in touch with his environment, fell from the third loft, and "was taken for dead." The good news is that Paul restored him to life—or maybe just woke him up. Eutychus must have been both grateful and embarrassed.

Sleep, or lack thereof, is an extremely important part of our life. By understanding more about sleep, you can make the necessary changes on your own—if you need to make any changes. At least 40 percent of Americans have sleep problems. You may be one of them, so keep reading.

When it comes to understanding sleep pathology, because of a unique experience, my interest in sleep has been heightened. Early in my sophomore year in medical school I volunteered for a "sleep study." The enticement was that each of the six of us who constituted the experiment cohort would receive $10 for the first sleepless 24 hours, $15 for the second sleepless period, and if we made it to the 72-hour mark of no sleep, the last reward was $25. Now, some babysitters I know get that in one night from tending two kids! But that was a lot of money then, and particularly with Christmas just around the corner.

All we had to do was stay awake and give blood and urine samples. We had monitors to keep notes and make sure we stayed awake. All sorts of crazy things happened to most of us as the hours dragged by. The last day, I remember looking at the linoleum floor, with squares arranged so that every other square was light, then dark, then light, and so forth. It looked to me as if the light squares were three to four inches higher than the dark squares, so I had to be careful walking so as not to trip. The terminal event (it felt very terminal) was to take the U.S. Army inductee questionnaire, given to those who were to wear the military uniform. We all failed! The good news was we did not qualify to be a part of our military force, but were allowed to remain in medical school. That tells you something about the intellect of sleep-deprived medical students.

The physiology of sleep can be characterized this way: to promote sleep, you have to block being awake, and to promote wakefulness, you have to block sleep. That is just how it is. We have an internal clock producing what we call the *circadian rhythm* and an external clock we call the *external extrinsic sleep drive*. Neither have anything to do with computers, as you will see.

After waking in the morning, you put both feet on the floor and head to the bathroom. However, you will not be fully awake until late morning. All of us work through this until we get our "second wind." The normal person is then ready for the remainder of the day, ideally a day full of opportunity and hope. The highest level of wakefulness occurs during late evening and the early part of the night. The build up of adenosine with a normal circadian rhythm can result in good sleep onset.

Studies show that peak athletic performance occurs in the late afternoon, and physical fitness scores at 2 p.m. are about 13 percent higher than those at 5 a.m. The word for wakefulness, as a sleep specialist may say, is vigilance. Good sleep will produce wakefulness and encourage vigilance. In my estimation, the purpose for sleep is to prepare you for the next day.

**What Sleep Does and Doesn't Do for Us**

Sleep maintains normal homeostatic processes. Brain neurochemistry and regulatory process repositioning occurs during sleep. Growth hormone is produced during sleep. In many organs, growth hormone aids repair of the tissues, and it's also involved in muscle mass maintenance. During sleep, there is a consolidation of new memories obtained during the day. The sleep process itself allows for injury repair, both to mind and body. The consensus is that the human body needs seven and a half to eight hours a night of sleep. Many physiologic studies show improved performance after seven hours of sleep. What does your sleep log show?

Sleep loss can come from a number of causes. There is not enough time or space to go into each of the causes of sleep loss, although admittedly, expounding on the causes may be more helpful than for me to list all the bad things that occur from sleep challenges. If you are able to identify the cause of your own sleep challenges, you may be able to handle them without a doctor's visit. But because sleep is so, so important, and because the cause or causes are so complex, see your physician if you can't get resolution to your problem. Having said that, many people have significant sleep problems and just don't know it. That is common.

Now, to the causes. Pets in bed, sleep apnea, a restless bed partner, alcohol, caffeine, medications, being overtired, late evening exercise, pain, depression, anxiety, gastroesophogeal reflux, shift work, an irregular sleep schedule, or lifestyle factors such as family conflicts, late night television, and internet mania.

Lets break down the adverse effects of sleep loss into acute sleep loss and chronic sleep loss.

## Effects of Acute Sleep Loss

Sleep-deprived individuals have a four- to six-fold increase in risk of death by motor vehicle accident. (This reminds me of the man who heard that 75 percent of the motor vehicle deaths occur within 15 miles of home, so he moved.) Response times are slowed, and there is a narrowed attention span, irritability, and cognitive impairment. As reported in Occupational and Environmental Medicine, published in 2000, a study showed that sleep deprivation affects cognitive performance equivalent or worse than a blood alcohol level of 0.05 percent.[227] I am sure you wouldn't drink and drive, but you may be one of the 40 percent who drives and without enough sleep. Your chance of injuring someone or yourself is greater, in this case, than if you drink alcohol and drive.

## Effects of Chronic Sleep Loss

Because of actual impairment of blood flow to the brain, and the resultant negative chemical interactions, we find cognitive impairment, decreased insight and awareness, and in general decreased quality of life in those who are sleep-deprived. All of this is a tremendous disadvantage when one wants to start the day with confidence and at the height of one's abilities. The list grows as it effects one's health: increased mortality due to cardiovascular (CV) disease, metabolic disease, diabetes, psychiatric disorders such as depression and anxiety, and increased weight gain. One study found that those who slept more than 7.7 hours a night had the lowest body mass index (BMI) and lowest risk for diabetes, while individuals who slept less than 6.5 hours a night gained, on average, an additional five pounds a year. Shift workers with insufficient sleep gained an additional seven pounds a year.[228] Here is a revelation that might be the eureka experience for you: you can bet that if you are obese you have a sleep problem, and if you have a sleep problem, you are probably overweight or obese.

Something that you may not be aware of is the idea of accumulated sleep deprivation. This is exactly what it sounds like: getting behind on the seven-and-a-half hour-a-night sleep routine. If, after a bad night, you try to make it up the next night, restoration to normal may not happen. Sleep debt is not easily normalized. One week of sleep debt results in a substantial number of mental lapses and underperformance of complex mental tasks. Recovery from years of accumulated sleep debt is next to impossible. Sleep loss has effects on the

---

[227] http://www.ncbi.nlm.nih.gov/books/NBK19958/

[228]

https://atrium.lib.uoguelph.ca/xmlui/bitstream/handle/10214/8199/Filion_A._Jordan_201407_MSc.pdf?sequence=1

physical: it causes reduction in endurance, accuracy, and strength. The longer you are awake, the slower you get.

A Stanford study looked at basketball players who slept for an average of 6.7 hours a night. The study increased their sleep time to 7.9 hours a night. That sounds like quite a feat. What were the results? Amazing—at least to me. They found that players ran faster and shot better, increasing their shooting percentage by 9 percent.[229] That is enough to win close ballgames. I wish my shooting percentage in life could improve by 9 percent because of several good nights' sleep.

An item that catches the eyes of most women is that sleep deprivation is linked to skin aging. Researchers at Cleveland's University Hospitals Case Medical Center found that sleep deprivation can increase signs of skin aging and additionally retards the skin's ability to recover after excessive exposure to the sun. Said Elma Baron, MD, director of the Skin Study Center at UH Case Medical Center, "We can add premature aging to the growing list of consequences of poor/inadequate sleeping habits."[230]

Last but not least, insufficient sleep is associated with higher rates of heart disease, strokes, and high blood pressure. Sleeping less than six and a half hours a night doubles the risk for high blood pressure. Loss of sleep also leads to endothelial damage (lining of the vessels).

BOTTOM LINE: Individuals with insufficient sleep die earlier and have poorer quality of life.

---

[229] http://www.audio-digest.org/pages/htmlos/summary.html?sub1=FP6207

[230] http://www.consultant360.com/exclusives/sleep-deprivation-linked-skin-aging

# SPIRITUALITY

Physicians, as scientists and healers, can look back as recently as yesterday and be pleased with some phenomenal changes in how we have cast out devils and stamped out disease among our afflicted.
Thomas Richards, MD, expounded:

*Our 'sin' is not that we have found ways to cast out demons and reduce physical suffering but rather that we have come to believe that the tools of scientific inquiry will provide an ultimate solution to our deepest and uniquely human concern-which, in my opinion, center around the search for the meaning of our lives and for our place in an infinite universe.*

*We must begin to shed our delusion that we are saving lives, for there is no life that can be saved from its ultimate fate. 'Saving' lives is the concern of artists and the clergy, not of scientists. What we are really doing is prolonging life and reducing physical suffering.*[231]

I find this to be quite thought provoking and marvelous at the same time.
I believe that the purpose of life is the Taj Mahal of our small village. As a medical community, our sole purpose is not, as some might suppose, to prolong this life. It is even more than improving the quality of that extended lifespan. It is to offer compassion and understanding and to serve as an example.
American Family Physician tells us: "More than 80 percent of Americans perceive religion as important and spirituality as an important adjunct to their lives. Spirituality is recognized as a factor that contributes to health in many persons. The concept of spirituality is found in all cultures and societies. It is expressed in an individual's search for ultimate meaning through participation in religion and/or belief in God, family, naturalism, rationalism, humanism, and the arts."[232]
One needs spirituality! I love the expression "The spiritually strong find a meaning in everything that they do." And how true that is. In order to take full advantage of our existence, we need to have meaning in the very small components in life.
In my practice, I have always taught that spirituality and the belief in a power greater than ours is important. I have treated and worked with both ends of the spectrum—the group who, as the scriptures state, are "yea of little faith" and

---

[231] http://www.consultantlive.com/articles/"preventive-medicine"-and-"road-hell"-readers-respond
[232] American Family Physician, Volume 86, number 6, September 25, 2012

those who are in daily partnership with a being greater than themselves.

Concerning health matters, important questions that we often ask ourselves are, "Why is this happening to me now? Will I die? Who will be with me when I die? What will happen to me after I die? Will my family survive my loss? Will I be remembered? Is there a God?" These questions teach us that there are many important things in the lives of others we were unaware of, yet need to be able to respond to.

The definition of spirituality is rather broad and difficult to nail down. It is defined by Oxford English Dictionary as "The quality or condition of being spiritual; attachment to or regard for things of the spirit as opposed to material or worldly interests."[233] This definition doesn't enlighten me much. Let's look at another definition, from Wiktionary: "Concern for that which is unseen and intangible, as opposed to physical or mundane."[234] For me, that too is a little wobbly. In trying to find a concise and at the same time understandable definition, I came up with National Cancer Institute's rendition of spirituality: "Having to do with deep, often religious feelings and beliefs, including a person's sense of peace, purpose, connection to others, and beliefs about the meaning of life."[235] That is more like it!

Elder Dallin H. Oaks tells us: "To be spiritually minded is to view and evaluate our experiences in terms of the enlarged perspective of eternity."[236]

Romans 8:5–6: "To be spiritual is life and peace."[237]

Spirituality is determined by personal outlook and priorities.

Where does the medical community stand when it comes to spirituality?

A group of deans and faculty of medical schools met to determine the key elements of a medical school curriculum. Their findings were published in The Association of American Medical Colleges (AAMC) Report I: Learning Objectives for Medical Student Education, Guidelines for Medical Schools. First and foremost, the report states that a physician should be altruistic: "Physicians must be compassionate and empathic in caring for patients.... In all of their interactions with patients, they must seek to understand the meaning of the patients' stories in the context of the patients' beliefs and family and cultural values. They must continue to care for dying patients even when disease-specific therapy is no longer available or desired."[238] Inherent in providing medical care to our patients, we physicians must also have a generous portion of spirituality.

Currently in the medical school curriculum, courses are required in matters pertaining to spirituality. Student education covers all aspects of history taking—

---

[233] http://www.oed.com

[234] http://en.wiktionary.org/wiki/spirituality

[235] http://www.cancer.gov/cancertopics/cancerlibrary/epeco/africanamericans/module16-AA/epeco-module16aa-spirituality-pdf

[236] https://www.lds.org/general-conference/1985/10/spirituality?lang=eng

[237] https://www.lds.org/scriptures/nt/rom/8.5-6?lang=eng#4

[238] https://webcampus.drexelmed.edu/professionalism/AAMCMedicalSchoolObjectivesProject.pdf

the physical, social, emotional, and spiritual.

Patients, in general, wish to discuss spirituality. A 2011 Gallup poll found that 91 percent of U.S. folks believe in God or a universal spirit, and 81 percent consider religion important. Another 40 percent use faith to cope with illness, and 25 percent of patients use prayer for healing each year.[239]

A study of 456 outpatients at six academic medical centers found that 33 percent expressed a desire for their physician to ask them about their religious beliefs, 19 percent wanted their physician to pray with them—and, in the case of dying patients, that number went up to 50 percent.[240]

Hospitalized patients, the elderly, and those with terminal illness often wish to share their beliefs and to have their physician pray for or with them. Spirituality in one's life not only gives us purpose, but gives meaning to death as well. As a physician, I have been fortunate to be a part of the "miracle of death," for indeed it is a miracle. It is the transition from life on this earth to a realm beyond, to a more restful existence.

Research studies have also addressed this issue. In a *USA Weekend* Faith and Health Poll, 65 percent of respondents felt that it was good for doctors to speak with them about their spiritual beliefs, yet only 10 percent said a doctor actually had.[241] I wonder why? Is it a matter of not enough time, an insensitivity to the patients' needs, incompetence on the physicians' part, lack of confidence in being able to approach the matter, or what?

The Joint Commission for Hospital Accreditation (JCAHO) now requires a patient undergo spiritual assessment upon hospital admission.

The benefits of spirituality and the studies to support this premise are many. American Family Physician: "Research studies demonstrate that up to 94 percent of hospitalized patients believe spiritual health is as important as physical health, and 40 percent use faith to cope with their illness."[242] Studies show us that people who have regular spiritual practices tend to live longer. This suggests that spirituality could be an important clinical goal.

A study that appeared in the *American Journal of Public Health* advances one of the possible mechanisms. A higher blood level of a substance called interleukin IL-6 is associated with an increased incidence of disease. They studied 1,700 older adults who attended church and found that they were half as likely to have elevated levels of interleukin IL-6. The theory is that religious involvement may offer better coping skills, a richer social support system, and the strength of personal values.[243]

Herbert Benson, MD, a cardiologist at Harvard School of Medicine, tells us that spiritual commitment tends to enhance recovery from illness and surgery. He

---

239 http://www.gallup.com/poll/147887/americans-continue-believe-god.aspx

240 MacLean CD, Susi B, Phifer N, et al. Patient preference for physician discussion and practice of spirituality. J Gen Intern Med. 2003;18(1):38–43

241 http://www.ncbi.nlm.nih.gov/pmc/articles/PMC1305900/

242 http://www.aafp.org/afp/2012/0915/p546.html

243 http://www.ncbi.nlm.nih.gov/pmc/articles/PMC1305900/

says, "People who don't worry as much tend to have better health outcomes. Maybe spirituality enables... people to worry less, to let go and live in the present moment." As a result of his understanding of spirituality, Benson finds that "10 to 20 minutes of meditation twice a day leads to decreased metabolism, decreased heart rate, decreased respiratory rate, and slower brain waves."[244] This practice had wide application, benefiting such clinical maladies as insomnia, anxiety, depression, and chronic pain. He calls this "the relaxation response."

Spirituality teaches us that the dying person will be in the loving presence of God or a higher power, that they would live on with their children and others they love, and that death is not the end but a passage.

**Philippians 3:20-21**
*But our citizenship is in heaven, and from it we await a Savior, the Lord Jesus Christ, who will transform our lowly body to be like his glorious body, by the power that enables him even to subject all things to himself.*

Related to spirituality is the power of hope and positive thinking. The role of a physician is more than just the basic things like taking a history, touching the patient to gain information, and prescribing a therapy. It is to be compassionate, "to suffer with." It is to help patients find meaning in life, in suffering, in facing the future with hope. Religion and spirituality form the foundation for all of these things.

I think we can be better physicians and true partners in our patients living and in their dying if we can truly listen to their hopes, their fears, and their beliefs and incorporate these beliefs into their therapeutic plans.

BOTTOM LINE: Spirituality is a way of life, not an occasional experience. It must be found where we live, rather than in those places we fondly hope to visit.

---

[244] http://www.ncbi.nlm.nih.gov/pmc/articles/PMC1305900/

# IT'S OVER, BUT IT HAS REALLY ONLY JUST BEGUN

In recent decades, medicine has advanced far beyond treating patients with leeches and using maggots to clean up dead tissue. It is a challenging science, but one with great personal rewards. In my career as a physician, I have been privileged to be involved in the lives of my patients beyond simple office visits, prescriptions for penicillin, and sewing up lacerations. I have wept with those who have lost friends and loved ones, shed tears of joy with parents as they experience the birth of a child, and worried and agonized over the threat of death or loss of independence to a patient. I have seen advances in medical care that caused me wonder and awe.

I thank my predecessors who have worked so hard for the knowledge I have been able to acquire through their efforts and their hard work in molding the physical, emotional, and spiritual into something that benefits mankind. And I thank anyone who is willing and able to have the determination and commitment to become a healthier and happier person. Honestly, one of the greatest thrills of my life has been having a patient return to the office having "grabbed the golden ring" and made positive behavioral changes pertaining to lifestyle.

Steinway pianos are built today the same way they were 161 years ago when Henry Steinway started his business. They are a fine work of art. The Steinway Model D Concert Grand sells for about $50,000. Scores of craftsmen and thousands of parts are required to produce one of these magnificent instruments. The ultimate in skill and workmanship is the rim-bending process — when 18 layers of hard-rock maple are bent around an iron press to create the shape of a Steinway grand. Henry Steinway himself developed and patented this process in 1878. Five coats of lacquer are applied, and then they go to work hand-rubbing to give the shine characteristic of the product.

Do you feel like you have been bent and polished — and what of that finished product? Do you now shine? I hope you have seen great changes, particularly in your knowledge and motivation to achieve your health goals.

If you have been diligent and read the entire book, or the better part it, I hope that you now want for yourself a better life, a healthier life, and one filled with happiness and fulfillment. You will reap what you have sown.

Found on the Hampden County Courthouse: "Obedience to law is liberty." Obedience to the laws of health also free one to take advantage of all of the God-given physical and mental aptitudes. Live well and enjoy!

Reading the information, accepting the challenges of the book, then doing what has been asked of you is nothing more and nothing less than the law of the harvest. Galatians 6:7: "For whatsoever a man soweth, that shall he also reap."

One must sow, having faith that with tilling and watering, a bountiful harvest will occur. Nonetheless, the rewards of a plentiful harvest are directly proportional to the effort put into the project. I have suggested that some rewards will take a season to bear fruit, so don't be impatient.

I've heard an interesting story about the law of the harvest, told by Keith Miller and Bruce Larson, authors of *The Edge of Adventure*—a book about harvesting that which you reap. In the Amargosa Desert in California, there stood a rundown hut. Nearby was a well, the only source of water for miles around. Attached to the pump was a tin baking powder can with a message inside, written in pencil on a sheet of brown wrapping paper. This was the message:

> *This pump is all right. I put a new sucker washer into it and it ought to last several years. But the washer dries out and the pump has got to be primed. Under the white rock I buried a bottle of water, out of the sun. There's enough water in it to prime this pump, but not if you drink some first. Pour in about 1/4 and let her soak to wet the leather. Then pour in the rest medium-fast and pump like your life depends on it. You'll get water. The well never has run dry. Have faith. When you get watered up, fill the bottle and put it back like you found it for the next feller.*
> *Signed,*
> *Desert Pete*[245]

The seed was the small container with the limited amount of water. The harvest was all the water one could drink. All one needed to do was to have faith—and take enough action—to bring about the desired result. Faith, action, and a little time, and that's about it.

The application is this: "Pour in the rest and pump like your life depends on it." Literally, your life does depend on your pouring into the pump (developing for yourself an effective healthy lifestyle program), and then you must pump like your life depends on it (apply yourself and do that which you know is best).

The "next feller" may be your brother, neighbor, associate at work, or just one of your fellow Americans who can see your example. You will affect that "next feller" by not passing onto others the burden of our ever-growing medical expenditures. Selections about lifestyle, as it results to health, affect all of us. We live in a society that is intertwined, and we are dependent on each other. What one person does or doesn't do, another person may feel.

The vast majority of us are the recipients of the actions of society to some degree. Look at the 17 percent GDP (gross domestic product) for healthcare. Look at the parking lots now occupied with more and more handicapped spaces. One of the greatest legacies we can leave to family, friends, and country is

---

[245] *The Edge of Adventure*, Keith Miller and Bruce Larson, Fleming H Revell Co; Revised edition (October 1991)

healthy living. But what a man *has*, he may be dependent upon others; what he *is*, rests with himself alone.

I am seriously wondering, if you have made it through this book, how you are feeling. Have you, to some degree, achieved the goals you wrote down in the beginning? Have you persevered, at least to some extent? Do you feel beaten down, or have you perhaps felt some of the refiner's fire? Do you feel good about what you have become? Do you feel liberated? Many questions, only you can answer.

I suspect you have come a long way in your quest for a healthier and indeed a happier life. I bet the question you asked yourself at the outset of this experience—"Can I really do this?"—has been answered in the affirmative. It was suggested in the introduction that you write a short biography about your present health status and asses your health goals. It is now time to rewrite that exercise and see what you have accomplished.

The following is written on the tomb of an Anglican Bishop in the Crypts of Westminster Abbey in London:

*When I was young and free and my imagination had no limits, I dreamed of changing the world. As I grew older and wiser, I discovered the world would not change, so I shortened my sights somewhat and decided to change only my country. But it, too, seemed immovable. As I grew into my twilight years, in one last desperate attempt, I settled for changing only my family, those closest to me; but alas, they would have none of it. And now as I lie on my deathbed, I suddenly realize: If I had only changed myself first, then by example I would have changed my family. From their inspiration and encouragement, I would then have been able to better my country and, I may have even changed the world.*

John Robbins:

*Our beauty does not come from dominating and conquering and winning. It comes from blessing and appreciating and loving. Our glory does not come from being right or being in charge. Our glory comes from being who we really are.*

Turning over the last page of this book ends what has turned out to be a very large project. I congratulate you on what you have done. You now will make a difference in your life. At this point it is up to you, no one else.

# RESOURCES

The intent of this book is to present scientific and sometimes not-so-scientific (in other words, anecdotal) information upon which you can make informed and hopefully accurate decisions about your health, lifestyle, and diet. The path you choose will lead you to a successful future.

This is where I exit and leave you to your own devices and creative thinking. In other words, the "how to" is left up to you. I have made suggestions throughout this book, and list below some resources such as books and online sources for your consideration. You can choose the diets, check the calories and nutrients, develop other options, if appropriate, and be the major leader in pursuit of your goals.

## ONLINE RESOURCES

### Fitnessbuilder
https://www.pumpone.com/fitnessbuilder

- Access to more than 900 workouts, 7,000 exercise images, and videos
- Appropriate for all fitness levels, from beginner to advanced
- App: https://itunes.apple.com/us/app/fitnessbuilder/id306287984?mt=8

### Checkyourhealth.org
Utah Department of Health

- Eat healthy—everything including packing your lunch
- Physical activity recommendations
- Health screenings
- Articles and news

### Whatscookingamerica.net

- Health, beauty, diet
- Receipts
- Newspaper columns

### Sparkpeople.com

- Food and fitness trackers
- Helps with goals
- Articles and videos

## Go4Life.nia.nih.gov

- Focuses on the older population
- Helps select and develop exercise programs, make plans, set goals, try activities, and monitor progress
- Free printed materials

## Choosemyplate.gov
The site is interactive and enables one to tailor a diet plan based on age, gender, and activity levels

- Weight management and calories
- Physical activities
- Tracker and other tools
- Printable materials
- Healthy eating tools

## Myfitnesspal.com
Nutritional and calorie database (tutorial video to learn the program)

- Free online site with a mobile app
- Remembers your favorite foods
- Manages each meal and shows all the nutrients and calories

## MyFood-A-Pedia
Free mobile tool from the U.S. Department of Agriculture

- Provides quick access to nutrition information, calorie, nutrients, etc.
- Good glycemic index calendar

## Fooducate

- Free, easy access to all foods with calories
- Mobile app available
- A mobile app that reads food bar codes

## BOOKS

For those who do not have access to the internet, there are a number of excellent resources which may be purchased at grocery or bookstores to give calorie and nutritional information about specific foods, diets, and lifestyles choices.

***The Living Heart Brand Names Shopper's Guide*** by Michael DeBakey,
A guide to healthy eating which includes breakdowns of the calories, fat, sodium, carbohydrates, and fiber in various foods

***Forks over Knives: The Plant-Based Way to Health***, edited by Gene Stone
Plant-based diet information and plant-based recipes

***Prevent and Reverse Heart Disease*** by Caldwell Esselstyn, Jr.
Studies on coronary heart disease, their treatment, and the results, along with plant-based diet recipes

***The China Study*** by Colin Campbell, and Thomas Campbell II
A monumental study of a Chinese population and the health benefits of eating a diet low in animal protein, and other plant-based recommendations

***The Miami Mediterranean Diet*** by Michael Ozner
Losing weight and lowering the risk of heart disease with the use of the Mediterranean diet

***Exercise & Physical Activity*** by the National institute on Aging
Governmental guidelines about regular exercise and physical activity

## MORE BOOKS

Weight reduction often includes counting calories, and there are some good calorie books available as well for those who don't have access to the Internet or mobile apps:

***The Calorie King, Calorie Fat, and Carbohydrate Counter*** by Allan Borushek

***The Complete Book of Food Counts*** by Corinne Netzer

***My Calorie Counter*** by Maureen Namkoong and Jennifer Sucov

***The Most Complete Food Counter*** by Jo-Ann Heslin